Green for Life

ALSO BY VICTORIA BOUTENKO

Raw Family (with the Boutenko family)
12 Steps to Raw Food
Raw Family Signature Dishes
Green Smoothie Revolution

Green
for Life

The Updated Classic on Green Smoothie Nutrition

VICTORIA BOUTENKO, MA

Foreword by A. William Menzin, MD

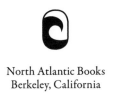

North Atlantic Books
Berkeley, California

Published by
North Atlantic Books
P.O. Box 12327
Berkeley, California 94712

Cover photo © istockphoto.com/lepas2004
Cover and book design by Claudia Smelser
Printed in the United States of America

First published in 2005 by Raw Family Publishing.

MEDICAL DISCLAIMER: The following information is intended for general information purposes only. Individuals should always see their health care provider before administering any suggestions made in this book. Any application of the material set forth in the following pages is at the reader's discretion and is his or her sole responsibility.

Green for Life is sponsored by the Society for the Study of Native Arts and Sciences, a nonprofit educational corporation whose goals are to develop an educational and cross-cultural perspective linking various scientific, social, and artistic fields; to nurture a holistic view of arts, sciences, humanities, and healing; and to publish and distribute literature on the relationship of mind, body, and nature.

North Atlantic Books' publications are available through most bookstores. For further information, visit our Web site at www.northatlanticbooks.com or call 800-733-3000.

LIBRARY OF CONGRESS CATALOGING-IN-PUBLICATION DATA
Boutenko, Victoria.
Green for life / by Victoria Boutenko ; foreword by
A. William Menzin.
p. cm.
Includes bibliographical references and index.
ISBN 978-1-55643-930-8
1. Nutrition. 2. Raw foods. 3. Smoothies (Beverages)
4. Cooking (Natural foods) I. Title.
RA784.B68   2010
613.2--dc22   2010027423

1 2 3 4 5 6 7 8 9 United 15 14 13 12 11 10

*I dedicate this book to Dr. Ann Wigmore
and all those who dare to think for themselves.*

ACKNOWLEDGMENTS

To my family, for always being extraordinarily dependable in all my endeavors, and for listening and discussing countless new concepts with me. To Dr. Paul Fieber and his wife, Susie, for their active help in organizing and conducting the Roseburg study. To all the participants of the Roseburg study for their time and commitment. To Vanessa Nowitzky for her quick fingers, impeccable grammar, and sweet sense of humor.

CONTENTS

FOREWORD

In more than thirty-five years of practice as a psychiatrist affiliated with the Harvard Medical School, I have learned one thing well: human behavior is very hard to change.

Now Victoria Boutenko is persuading me otherwise, because this remarkable woman has developed a strategy for helping ordinary Americans (the ones who love ice cream and steak and French fries and pizza) introduce green living foods into their life in a delicious and habit-forming way. Nothing she says in this book about our body's ability to restore itself to good health if given the right nutrients to work with is exactly new in itself. And yet *Green for Life* is a groundbreaking achievement because Ms. Boutenko has understood that the way to encourage her readers to trigger their natural mechanisms for cleaning cholesterol, fat, and toxins from their bodies—and thereby to improve first their physical lives and then their mental and spiritual lives—is not to lecture about the need to consume more living plant life but to make it easy and pleasant for them to do it.

The green smoothie—or, to be more specific, the quart of green smoothie that Ms. Boutenko recommends we all start our day with—is in and of itself a tremendous injection of chlorophyll, vitamins, minerals, enzymes, and antioxidants into the typical American diet. A quart of green smoothie a day also discourages consumption of denatured and greasy foods. For one thing, it's hard to stuff yourself with refined starches and sugars when you're full of one of Ms. Boutenko's tasty and energizing concoctions. (Check out one of the tempting recipes for Sweet Green Smoothies on page 176.) And if another seductive green smoothie is waiting for you in the refrigerator when you get home from work, the dinner you prepare and consume after sipping it will almost certainly be smaller, and possibly healthier, too.

Thirty days of green smoothies will also change how you feel and how you feel about yourself. That's no small achievement for one small book.

I salute Ms. Boutenko. I recommend that you take *Green for Life* very seriously. I believe it can help you change your life.

A. William Menzin, MD
Department of Psychiatry
Harvard Medical School
Former consultant to the World Health Organization (WHO)

Dear Reader,

I am flattered that *Green for Life* has become so popular and am honored to present you with this updated version of my book. Since it was first published, some major discoveries in the field of nutrition have occurred that I wanted to share with you. Of particular importance are several groundbreaking studies recently published about the proper balance of essential fatty acids. This new edition of *Green for Life* contains a whole new chapter about omega-3 oils; I believe these findings to be nearly as valuable as the entire concept of green smoothies themselves.

I am amazed at the speed with which the pool of nutritional information is growing. Many new discoveries about greens, fruits, and vegetables have recently appeared in scientific publications and throughout the Internet. When I was gathering information for my book back in 2004, there was almost no data available about greens. The only "green" that had nutritional analysis was cooked spinach. I had to search for pieces of information all over the world. Now the USDA provides comprehensive nutritional data on the majority of foods, including uncommon items such as stinging nettles, dandelions, and other weeds. In this updated edition I am pleased to include valuable new information on the nutritional content of some of my green smoothies and about several greens, fruits, and vegetables.

Another big chunk of important research came from thirty-seven new studies comparing the nutritional content of organic versus conventional foods; thus I felt the need to update the chapter about organic soil.

Finally, the latest research about the vital importance of antioxidant flavonoids in the human diet inspired me to create several new recipes, such as Minti-Dandelion and Super Cilantro, with more colorful ingredients rich in antioxidants.

Several powerful new testimonials about the healing potential of green smoothies further enhance this new edition.

I would like to thank my readers all over the world for their ongoing interest in natural health. All I did was write the book. You are the ones who change your health—and I celebrate with you!

In Health,
Victoria

INTRODUCTION

Dear Reader,

I am delighted to share this book with you. In the following chapters I disclose many astonishing facts about greens and explain why they are the most essential part of human nutrition. Ever since I realized the key to radiant health was under my very nose, I began to read every book on greens I could get my hands on.

Initially, I only wanted to improve the classic raw food diet. Surprisingly, in the process of my research, I found that adding blended greens to anyone's diet makes such a profound health improvement that it may even surpass the benefits of eating a typical all-raw diet with a relatively small amount of greens. In addition, drinking smoothies is far more doable than switching at once to an all-raw diet. At the same time, I have discovered that people who incorporate blended greens into their daily meals naturally begin to eat more live foods.

Blended green smoothies are a simple and delicious way of accessing the healing properties of greens. Whether you eat a raw food, vegan, vegetarian, or mainstream American diet, regularly drinking green smoothies can significantly improve your health. This miraculous drink is available to every person in every country. Join me in discovering why greens are the perfect human food. I hope this information is as refreshing for you as it has been for me.

—Victoria Boutenko

Dare to Observe!

Doubt is the father of invention.
—GALILEO GALILEI

Observation constitutes the foundation of every science. You and I, like everyone on this planet, have the right to make observations and draw our own conclusions, whether we are scientists or not. Our personal experimentation helps us stay in charge of our own lives. No scientific data can substitute for our own experience.

When a child is told not to touch the fire, this warning doesn't mean much until he or she actually tries touching the flames and gets hurt. Only through observation can we learn to connect consequences with causes, to become aware of what to expect. For example, if we overeat late at night, we should not expect to feel fresh in the morning. The advantage of being aware of what is going to happen enables us to act deliberately in our everyday lives and to achieve the goals we desire through conscious actions instead of constantly and blindly following the advice of somebody "who knows better."

I was raised in the Soviet Union, where everyone was severely controlled by the government structures. From early childhood I was given firm instructions about what I was supposed to do, say, and even think. I was afraid to try anything new. However, I was very lucky to meet many incredible people in my life from whom I learned to dare to try everything I wanted.

I absolutely have to tell you about Alexander Suvorov, whom I met several times and who became my hero and inspiration for many years. Suvorov became totally blind and deaf when he was three years old. Nevertheless, he was so eager to live his life to the fullest that he learned to speak and to understand what other people were saying by holding their hands. He graduated from high school with honors and acquired a PhD at Moscow University. Suvorov wrote dozens of brilliant books on philosophy and countless scientific articles about helping blind and deaf children. While being unable to view a single movie himself, Suvorov created three engaging documentaries about his perception of life. I recall the presentation of his first film. It attracted huge crowds in Moscow in the 1970s. People were deeply impressed by Suvorov's sincerity and passion. I remember that after the movie was over, nobody left the theater for a long time. We just sat there bewildered, sobbing, and ashamed of our cowardly lives and stupid fears. Alexander Suvorov, living his life in physical darkness and constant silence, had a dream to travel to other countries. So he learned two foreign languages and traveled to several countries on his own. When people asked him why he went, he replied that he wanted "to see the world for himself."

When I meet incredible human beings like Suvorov or read about people who dare to "see for themselves," I begin to want to explore life around me in more depth and find out how far my limits can stretch.

As we live our lives, trying new things and searching for true answers, we gain plenty of our own experiences. Our knowledge becomes familiar and practical. We feel rather confident in any life circumstance, particularly when we need to make urgent decisions. Contrary to that, when all we have is a compilation of someone else's instructions, the best we can do is to hope and pray that the authors of such instructions were efficient in acquiring their knowledge and honest in their intentions. In other words, we hope that someone else cares for us more than we care for ourselves.

When we let others observe and reason for us, in a sense we consciously choose to stay blind and deaf. We become compelled to follow someone else's instructions, one after another, and perform actions that do not make much sense to us. We submit to the authority of others. We give our power away.

To observe is our birthright. If we utilize our ability to observe, we can free ourselves from the labyrinth of confusions. I believe that our own conscious observations are a thousand times more important than any rigid scientific claim.

Why have so many books on nutrition been published of late? Obviously there is a big question from the public about health that has not been satisfied by the scientific wing of our world community. Most of us are totally cut off from researchers, and at the same time, scientists are disconnected from ordinary people. I wonder why this has happened, since the original goal of science is human well-being.

Most results of pure science are unavailable and unaffordable for common people. For example, in order to obtain a two- or three-page report of a medical study I had to pay a lot of money, sometimes hundreds of dollars for each one. The average research paper is written in complex scientific terms, which makes it incomprehensible to people who don't belong to that particular branch of science. I have observed that the branches of science are increasing in number and the language they use continually multiplies in terminology. Throughout my life I have spoken to dozens of different scientists in different parts of the world, and I have never met one scientist who was able to understand and explain studies from all the branches at the same time. In fact, the more scientists claim to know about one subject, the more they tend to say, "That's not my field," about the others.

This tendency suggests that science is moving beyond the understanding of the average person toward science for the sake of science. While the public wants to know about the newest achievements, the scientific world becomes less and less available to answer their burning questions. An information vacuum begins to grow, especially in the field of health and nutrition.

To substitute for this missing yet crucial information, the public begins to conduct its own research, which may not be completely accurate but is understandable to the majority of people. Hence, we witness hundreds if not thousands of books on nutrition written by average people who undertake different research studies, sometimes without the necessary background. Desperate for answers to their questions, people absorb this abundance of information and often get more confused.

I notice that many people trust the written word more than the spoken word. Due to the lack of people's own observations and a tendency to believe whole concepts as if they were set in stone, health seekers embrace a certain concept, often depending on which book they have read first. As multitudes of nutritional books are generated, they begin to contradict one another. As a result, it is possible to encounter hundreds of people today with completely different suggestions for what to eat, all with hundreds of different reasons that cancel each other out.

When I started to do research about greens, I instantly and hopelessly sank into an ocean of information. In my situation *I had to find the true answer or die.* I felt responsible not only for my husband and my children, whom I had dragged onto the raw food diet with me, but for all those thousands of people in the world that I inspired to adopt an all-raw diet. Finally, I decided to put everything aside for several months to sit down and read through as many original research papers as I could get on the subject of nutrition. I decided to cut away all the opinions and focus only on the original data because human reasoning can build up logical chains of thought that smoothly direct the reader to totally incorrect conclusions with devastating results. (Later in this book, I will give examples of such mistakes in which I myself got trapped.)

I discovered that there were some substantial gaps in the data, including numerous important foods whose properties have never been studied. I realized that if I wanted to draw the right conclusions, I had to initiate at least some pilot studies by myself. After all, my life was already an experiment in which I was the guinea pig.

I strongly believe, now more than ever, that it is safer to go on raw food for two weeks to see for yourself how you feel than to read ten books and follow their recommendations without having any idea why. Through our careful observations we all have the ability to clearly see the results of our actions.

Dear reader, with this book I hope to inspire you to start observing which of your actions makes you feel and look the healthiest, and as a result to create a personal plan that will work for you in the best way. You are your own best expert.

2

What Was Missing in Our Raw Food Plan?

My husband, our two youngest children, and I have been eating a raw food diet since January 1994. We went on this radical diet out of complete despair when our medical doctors couldn't offer us any means to recover from our horrible illnesses.

My husband, Igor, had been constantly ill since his early childhood. By the age of seventeen he had already survived nine surgeries. Having progressive hyperthyroidism and chronic rheumatoid arthritis, at thirty-eight he was a total health wreck. I had to lace his shoes on rainy days because his arthritic spine would not bend. Igor's heart rate was 140-plus most of the time, his eyes were tearing on sunny days, and his hands were shaky. Igor constantly felt fatigued and was in pain almost all the time. Igor's thyroid doctor told him that he would die in less than two months if he would not agree to have his thyroid gland removed. His arthritis doctor told him to prepare to spend the rest of his life in a wheelchair.

I was diagnosed with the same disease that took my father: arrhythmia, or an irregular heartbeat. My legs were constantly swollen from edema, I weighed 280 pounds, and I was continuously gaining more weight. My left arm frequently became numb at night and I was afraid that I would die and my children would become orphans. I remember always feeling tired and depressed.

Our daughter Valya was born with asthma and allergies and would often cough heavily all through the night. Our son Sergei was diagnosed with diabetes.

One day, after crying through the entire night, I decided that we had to take a *different* action if we wanted to get *different* results. That was when we started to try various healing modalities and eventually arrived at the idea of becoming raw foodists. At the time we didn't know anything about making fancy raw dishes or even that we could dehydrate our own flax crackers. Nevertheless, by turning off the pilot light in our stove and discontinuing all cooking, we were able to heal all of our "incurable" life-threatening diseases. Our health was improving so quickly that in three and a half months all four of us ran the Bolder Boulder 10K race with forty thousand other runners.

Even Sergei's blood sugar stabilized due to his new diet and regular jogging. Since beginning to eat raw food, he has never again experienced any form of diabetic symptoms. We were greatly surprised not only by how quickly our health was restored to normal but by how much healthier we were than ever before. We have described the detailed story of our miraculous healing in our book *Raw Family: A True Story of Awakening.*

After several years of being raw foodists, however, each one of us began to feel like we had reached a plateau where our healing process stopped and even began to go somewhat backward. After approximately seven years on a completely raw diet, once in a while, and then more and more frequently, we started feeling discontent with our existing food program. I began to get a heavy feeling in my stomach after eating almost any kind of raw food, especially a salad with dressing. Because of that, I started to eat fewer greens and more fruits and nuts. I began to gain weight. My husband started to develop a lot of gray hair. My family members felt confused about our diet and often seemed to have the question, "What should we eat?" There were odd times when we felt hungry but did not desire any of the foods that were "legal" for us to eat on a typical raw food diet: fruits, nuts, seeds, grains, or dried fruit. Salads (with dressings) were delicious but made us tired and sleepy. We felt trapped. I remember Igor looking inside the fridge, saying over and over again, "I wish I wanted some of this stuff." Such periods did not last. At first we blamed it all on overeating and were able to refresh our appetites by fasts, hikes or other exercise, or by working more. In my family we strongly believed that *raw food was the only way to go,* and therefore we encouraged each other to maintain our raw diet no matter what, always coming up with new tricks. Many of my friends told me about similar experiences, at which point they gave up being one-hundred-percent raw and began to add cooked food back into their meals. In my family, we continued to stay on raw food due to our constant support of each other.

A burning question began to grow stronger in my heart with each day. The question was, "Is there anything missing in our diet?" The answer would come right away: "Nope. Nothing could be better than a raw food diet."

Yet, the unwanted signs of less-than-perfect health, however tiny, kept surfacing in minor but noticeable symptoms such as a wart on a hand or a gray hair, which brought doubts and questions about the completeness of the raw food diet, at least in its present form. Finally, when my children complained about the increased sensitivity of their teeth, I reached a state where I couldn't think about anything besides this health puzzle. I drove everybody around me crazy with my constant discussion of what could possibly be missing.

In my eager quest, I started collecting data about every single food that existed for humans. As my grandmother used to say, "Seek and ye shall find." After many wrong guesses, I finally found the correct answer. I found one particular food group that matched *all* human nutritional needs: greens. The truth is, in my family, we were not eating enough greens. Moreover, we did not like them. We knew that greens were important, but we never heard anywhere exactly what quantity of greens we needed in our diet. We had only a vague recommendation to eat as much of them as possible. In order to find out how many greens we needed to eat, I decided to find an animal that was genetically closest to humans. All research pointed to chimpanzees, which share an estimated 99.4 percent of their genes with humans.

3

How Chimpanzees Eat

Chimpanzees are very similar to humans. Scientists at the Chimpanzee and Human Communication Institute at Washington Central University believe that "chimpanzees should be categorized as a people."[1] For after closely studying the behavior of these intelligent beings, the researchers at WCU have become convinced that chimpanzees are significantly smarter than most people think. According to these scientists, chimpanzees have their own language and culture that humans didn't even suspect they possessed, probably because chimpanzees do not speak. They do, however, use their own sign language, which scientists have been studying closely for almost four decades. The researchers at WCU stated:

> New evidence indicates that the technology and the communication of the chimpanzee community meets the definition of culture. We also know that chimpanzee's cognitive capacities are very similar to our own, both intellectually and emotionally. By any reasonable definition *chimpanzees should be categorized as a people.*[2]

Most medical research institutes agree that chimpanzees and humans are very alike. Unfortunately, based on this fact, they use chimpanzees in scientific experiments. Take a look at the following quotes from various medical articles.

Modern people and chimpanzees share an estimated 99.4% of our DNA sequence, making us more closely related to each other than either is to any other animal species.[3]

Chimpanzees resemble humans more than any other animal. ... Human brains are very like chimpanzee brains. The major differences between humans and apes are not anatomical, but rather behavioral.[4]

Chimps have the same A-B-O blood groupings as humans and are used for compatibility studies for tissue transplants, for hepatitis research, and for other medical studies.[5]

Nonhuman primates [play a] critical role in biomedical research of understanding, treatment, and prevention of important infectious diseases such as AIDS, hepatitis, and malaria, and chronic degenerative disorders of the central nervous system (like Parkinson's and Alzheimer's diseases). ... The close phylogenetic relation of NHPs to humans not only opens avenues for testing the safety and efficacy of new drugs and vaccines but also offers promise for evaluating the potential of new gene-based treatments for human infectious and genetic diseases.[6]

Nonhuman primates are excellent models for studying human biology and behavior because of their close phylogenetic relation to humans. Their use in biomedical research is critical to advancements in medical science ... [including] the discovery of the Rh factor and the development of the poliovirus vaccine. ... Their use has expanded into virtually every area of medicine.[7]

If chimpanzees and humans were really so closely related, and studying this closeness was so critical to our health, I wondered, *why don't we humans apply our studies both ways?* How could it be that we foist our worst human illnesses on chimpanzees but we don't learn from them? Rather than making them sick, why not make ourselves well? Why not at least try out what they eat?

I went online and purchased $300 worth of books and DVDs about chimpanzees and their diet and lifestyle. I wrote a letter with my questions to Jane Goodall's university. I traveled to three big zoos that have chimpanzees and spoke to many people who feed them and take care of them every day. While visiting Russia, I had an opportunity to spend several days observing and participating in the feeding process with the chimps that lived at the Moscow Circus. I discovered fascinating information about chimpanzees that totally changed my view of them.

I was very impressed to find out that chimpanzees can learn to use human sign language:

Under double-blind conditions, we have found that the chimpanzees communicate information in American Sign Language (ASL) to human observers. They use signs to refer to natural language categories: e.g. *dog* for any dog, *flower* for any flower, *shoe* for any shoe, etc. The chimpanzees acquire and spontaneously use their signs to communicate with humans and each other about the normal course of surrounding events. They have demonstrated an ability to invent new signs or combine signs to metaphorically label a novel item, for example: calling a radish *cry hurt food* or referring to a watermelon as a *drink fruit*. In a double-blind condition, the chimpanzees can comprehend and produce novel prepositional phrases, understand vocal English words, translate words into their ASL glosses, and even transmit their signing skills to the next generation without human intervention. Their play behavior has demonstrated that they use the same types of imaginary play as humans. It has also been demonstrated that they carry on chimpanzee-to-chimpanzee conversation and sign to themselves when alone. Conversational research shows the chimpanzees initiate and maintain conversations in ways that are like humans. The chimpanzees can repair a conversation if there is misunderstanding. They will also sign to themselves when alone, and we have even observed them to sign in their sleep.[8]

When I educated myself about chimpanzees, they became one of my favorite beings. Understanding their intelligent nature, I feel deeply sorry for the 1,500 chimps that spend their lives in tiny indoor cages in medical laboratories in the United States.

Despite all the scientific research, human health continues to decline. Many nutritionists connect human health problems with nutritional deficiencies. Humans have lost their natural way of eating. That is why I am so grateful that there is another species in this world that closely resembles us. In particular, I was glad to know that there are thousands of chimpanzees living in the Gombe Valley in East Africa. Remarkably, the majority of the chimps of Gombe, unlike humans, have not been touched by civilization. This is very fortunate for us humans, as it gives us hope to find the answers to our most vital questions: What is the human diet supposed to be? What was it originally? If we share 99.4 percent of the same genes with chimpanzees, it is logical to hypothesize that our diets are supposed to be 99.4 percent similar.

Understanding chimpanzees' eating habits may help us better understand human dietary needs. Look at this chart showing the average diet of the chimpanzee in the wilderness. I created this chart based on data from Jane Goodall's books:

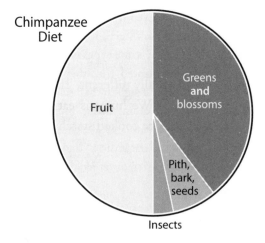

Chimpanzee Diet

Fruit

Greens and blossoms

Pith, bark, seeds

Insects

As you can see, the two major food groups for chimpanzees are fruits and greens. It's important not to confuse greens with root vegetables like carrots, beets, or potatoes, or with nonsweet fruits like cucumbers, tomatoes, zucchini, and bell peppers. Chimps rarely eat root vegetables, and they do so primarily in cases of drought or famine as a fallback food.[9] According to Jane Goodall, the world-famous researcher of chimpanzees, the amount of greens that chimpanzees eat in relation to the rest of their diet varies from 25 to 50 percent, depending on the season.[10] Between 2 and 7 percent of their diet is pith and bark. (Pith is the stems and more fibrous parts of plants.) When the trees are blooming, in March and April, chimpanzees consume blossoms, which comprise up to 10 percent of their diet. Chimpanzees do not eat very many nuts, but their diet could be up to 5 percent seeds. They also consume small amounts of insects and even small animals, particularly in November. However, Goodall says this part of their diet is irregular and insignificant as chimpanzees can go many months without eating any animals and seem to suffer no ill effects.

For as long as I can remember, chimpanzees have been depicted with a banana or an orange in their hands, which definitely misled me to the assumption that they eat only fruit. To know that greens compose almost half of their diet was a revelation for me. My research gave me a solid understanding that humans are supposed to eat far more greens than I would have guessed.

Let's compare the standard American diet with that of the chimpanzee diet. As you can see, they look totally different. These two diets have hardly anything in common! We humans eat mostly things that chimpanzees don't eat at all, like cooked starchy foods, oils, butter, yogurt, cheese, and hamburgers. While most of our vegetables are roots, wild chimpanzees almost never eat root vegetables unless fruits and greens are unavailable. It is the intake of greens that has declined most dramatically in the human diet. Our consumption of greens has generally shrunk to the two wilted iceberg lettuce leaves on our sandwich.

Let's compare the standard American diet with the diet of a typical raw foodist.

I think that a raw food diet demonstrates a vast improvement over the regular American diet. Firstly, all ingredients in a raw diet are uncooked and full of enzymes and vitamins; thus the raw food diet is like a revolution in comparison with the standard American diet. That explains why so many people have reported that they instantly felt better when they began a raw diet. We can see that raw foodists eat a lot of fruit, especially if we keep in mind that bell peppers, cucumbers, zucchini, and tomatoes are also fruits. However, even though raw foodists typically consume many more greens than people on an average mainstream diet do, greens rarely constitute 45 percent of their food. So what do raw foodists eat in place of their missing greens? Most consume large amounts of fruits, nuts, and seeds. Often they use nuts as a substitute for carbohydrates, particularly when trying to mimic cooked dishes with raw ingredients, even though nuts are 70–80 percent fat. Also, raw foodists increase their consumption of oils and avocados because the most common way of eating salad, their main staple, is to mix it with dressing, sauce, or guacamole. Another big part of a typical raw diet is root vegetables, mostly used in juicing. Also, roots taste sweeter than greens and thus comprise a large portion of raw salads.

Considering all these factors, when we compare the typical raw food diet with the chimpanzee diet, we can clearly see that there are two main ways to improve our eating patterns further: to increase our consumption of greens and to reduce our intake of nuts, seeds, and oils.

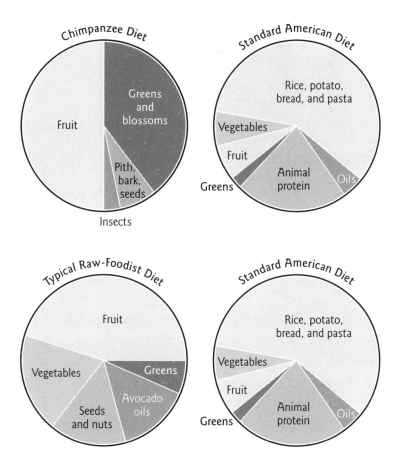

To calculate how many greens we needed to consume in my family, I looked at how much fruit we consumed. At about four or five pounds of fruit per day per person, I estimated that we needed to eat one to two good-sized bunches of dark leafy greens per person per day, or one to two pounds.

Another striking aspect of the chimpanzee eating pattern is that they never eat in the late afternoon or evening. Chimpanzees wake up very early, at the first light of dawn. After leaving their nests they groom each other for a few minutes and then begin searching for food. Chimpanzees have to work hard in order to get their food,

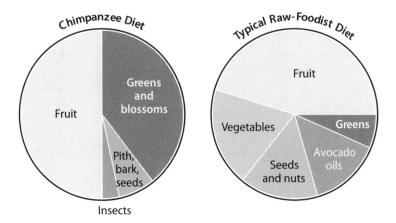

climbing many trees or searching through numerous low shrubs. Most often they feed on fruit in the morning and a little bit on leaves. After about four hours, they take a break for an hour or two, playing or sleeping in the sun. Then the chimps resume feeding, eating mostly greens until about 3 or 4 o'clock in the afternoon, after which they groom and prepare their nests for the night's sleep.

In contrast, my own eating pattern is vastly different. I don't normally eat anything until noon or later, and in the evening I stock up on food. I am currently striving to stop eating after 6 p.m. While I am experiencing positive results and finally shedding some extra weight, I have to admit that restraining myself from eating late is a lot harder than I expected. I attribute this to the larger amount of stress we tend to accumulate towards the end of the day.

4

Green Smoothie Revolution

In my research I noticed that chimpanzees *love* greens. I remember watching chimps at the zoo and seeing how excited they became when given fresh acacia branches, young tender palm tree leaves, or kale. Looking at them, I was so inspired that I went to the nearby bushes and tried to eat acacia leaves myself. But the green leaves were not very palatable for me, and that presented another problem: eating greens always seemed like a duty for me. I would think to myself, *I have to eat my greens.* Some days I would "cheat" by juicing my greens. I would quickly drink a cup of green juice and consider myself good for a couple of days. Or, before I gave up oils, I would enjoy my greens by making a delicious raw dressing and sinking them into it. But I could never imagine sitting down and eating a bunch of kale or spinach.

While I disliked greens, my husband, Igor, simply couldn't tolerate them. When he was growing up he was encouraged to eat mostly meat and bread, "like a real Russian man." Living in Russia, we rarely saw any greens in stores. People could buy dill, parsley, and green onions at farmers markets, but only in the summer. I recall seeing lettuce about twice each summer and considered it rare and exotic.

The more I read about the nutritional content of greens, the more I became convinced that greens were the most important food for humans. If only I could find a way to enjoy them enough to consume the quantity needed to become perfectly healthy!

Countless times I tried to force myself to eat large amounts of greens in the form of salad or by themselves, only to discover that I was not physically able to do so. After about two cups of shredded greens I would either have heartburn or nausea.

One day, while reading a book on biology, I became intrigued by the amazingly hardy composition of plants. Apparently cellulose, the main constituent of plants, has one of the strongest molecular structures on the planet. Greens possess more valuable nutrients than any other food group, but all these nutrients are stored inside the cells of the plants. These cells are made of tough material, probably as a means of survival for the plant, to make it difficult for animals to eat. To release all the valuable nutrients from within the cells, the cell walls need to be ruptured, but breaking through these sturdy cells is not easy. This is why eating greens without chewing them thoroughly does not satisfy our nutritional needs. We need to chew our greens to a creamy consistency in order to get their benefits.

In addition, to digest the released minerals and vitamins, the hydrochloric acid in the stomach has to be very strong, with a pH between 1 and 2.

These two conditions are absolutely, vitally necessary for the assimilation of nutrients from greens. Obviously, when I tried to eat plain greens I did not chew them well enough and possibly did not have a high enough level of hydrochloric acid in my stomach. As a result, I experienced unpleasant signs of indigestion and developed a general dislike for greens altogether.

After many decades of eating heavily processed foods, most of us have lost our ability to chew normally.[1] Our jaws have become so narrow that most of us need to wear braces because there is simply not enough space for all of our teeth, even if our wisdom teeth have been extracted.[2] Our jaw muscles have become too weak to chew rough fiber thoroughly. Several times my dentist has urged me to be gentler on my teeth, and not to bite firm fruits and vegetables but rather to grate my carrots and apples. Many people also have lots of fillings, false teeth, or missing teeth. All of these obstacles make chewing greens to the necessary consistency virtually impossible.

This is why I decided to try to "chew" my greens using a Vita-Mix blender.* First I blended a bunch of kale with water. I was thinking, *I will just close my eyes and nose and drink it.* But as soon as I opened the lid, I quickly closed it again because I felt queasy from the strong wheatgrass smell. That dark green, almost black, mixture was totally unconsumable. After some brainstorming, I added several bananas and blended it again. And that was when the magic began. Slowly and with some trepidation, I removed the lid and sniffed the air, and to my great surprise, this bright green concoction smelled very pleasant. I was so anxious to try it that I began drinking it right from the blender. I cautiously tasted a sip and was exhilarated—it was better than tasty! Not too sweet, not too bitter, it was the most unusual taste I had ever experienced, and I could describe it in one word: freshness.

In four hours, I had consumed everything I had blended, which was one bunch of kale, four bananas, and a quart of water. I felt wonderful and made more. Triumphantly, I realized that this was the

---

*Vita-Mix is not like the blenders you can find at any department store. It is called a high-speed blender because its motor reaches speeds of up to 240 miles per hour. That means that the blades don't have to be sharp; even if they were just dull metal sticks they could still liquefy something as hard as blocks of wood. In order to reach such performance, the Vita-Mix has a 2+ peak horsepower motor. Most other blenders will blend the tough cellulose of greens only as long as their blades are sharp. When the blades become dull, they just move food pieces around and the blender very quickly overheats. Fifteen years ago, after burning out several blenders, I finally bought myself a Vita-Mix at the county fair. It still works like new. I promote this blender because in my experience, it is the best I have found. You can purchase a Vita-Mix at www.rawfamily.com.

first time in my life that I had consumed two good-sized bunches of greens in one day. Plus I ate them without any oil or salt and I enjoyed the whole experience. My stomach felt fine, and I was overjoyed to have achieved my goal.

That was in August 2004. The solution to my greens dilemma was unexpectedly simple. To consume greens in this way took so little time that I naturally continued experimenting with blended greens and fruits day after day.

I must admit here that the idea of blended greens was not new to me. Sixteen years ago when my family was studying at the Creative Health Institute (CHI) in Michigan, we were taught about the extraordinary healing properties of energy soup: blended sprouts, avocado, and apple. This soup was invented by Dr. Ann Wigmore, the pioneer of the living-foods lifestyle in the twentieth century. Although we were told countless times how exceptionally beneficial energy soup was, most of the guests at the institute were not able to eat more than a couple of spoonfuls of energy soup because it was not palatable.

I was very impressed with the testimonials that I heard from people about the benefits of energy soup. When I returned home I desperately experimented with energy soup, trying to improve the taste because I wanted my family to benefit from eating it. My final attempt to perfect energy soup was ended one day when I heard Valya yelling to Sergei in the back yard, "Run! Mom is making that green mush again!"

Despite all the evidence of the healing powers of energy soup, I found that, unfortunately, even people who desperately needed and wanted it could not make themselves consume it regularly.

I am amazed that many years after being introduced to energy soup, when I had completely forgotten all about it, I came back to the very same idea of blended greens from an entirely new direction. When I first started drinking green smoothies, I did not expect anything significant to happen. Although I didn't have any serious health problems, I did hope to find a way to cure the nagging ailments my family and I were experiencing. After about a month of erratic green smoothie drinking, two moles and a wart I'd had since early childhood peeled off my body. I felt more energized than ever before and started sharing my experience with my family and friends. The next thing I noticed was that those cravings I had occasionally for heavy foods such as nuts or crackers, especially in the evenings, had totally disappeared. I noticed that many of the wrinkles on my face went away and I began to hear compliments from other people about my fresh look. My nails became stronger, my vision sharpened, and I had a wonderful taste in my mouth, even upon waking in the morning (a pleasure I hadn't had since youth).

My dream had come true at last! I was consuming plenty of greens every day. I began to feel lighter and my energy increased. My tastes started to change. I discovered that my body was so starved for greens that for several weeks I lived almost entirely on green smoothies. Plain fruits and vegetables became much more desirable to me and my cravings for fatty foods declined dramatically. I stopped consuming any kind of salt altogether.

Two weeks later, my husband and I were walking along a trail in California covered with succulent chickweed and dandelions when I suddenly noticed that I was salivating. The dark-green weeds growing in abundance along our path looked so scrumptious. I kept catching myself wanting to grab and eat them. I shared my observations with Igor; he listened attentively but didn't get excited. He had already noticed that I was eating differently lately. Instead of making myself a huge salad of several chopped vegetables, a large avocado, sea salt, lots of onion, and olive oil, I now chopped up a bunch of lettuce with a tomato, sprinkled it with lemon juice, and enjoyed it tremendously, rolling my eyes and humming with pleasure. I did not miss my former food and felt completely satisfied eating simply. I had learned for sure that the human body can learn to crave greens.

There was another change that astounded me. I used to have cravings for unhealthy foods when I got tired. For example, in the past, when I was traveling and would spend the night on an airplane, or after driving all night, I experienced severe cravings for some heavy raw foods or even for some authentic Russian cooked foods from my childhood that I hadn't eaten in more than a decade. These cravings were very strong and annoying. Driven by these urges, I would prepare myself some kind of dense raw food like seed cheese with crackers or stuff myself with nuts, sometimes late at night. I have heard from many other people that they experienced similar patterns. Also, during previous years, when I came home late from my office, often after 10 p.m., I enjoyed changing my focus from work to other lighter topics, either by reading a chapter in a book or by watching a nice video. I noticed that if I allowed myself to grab an apple or a handful of nuts, I would tend to continue grazing and couldn't ever achieve a feeling of satisfaction. Even if I used my willpower and didn't touch any food at home, I continued to feel discontent and food kept coming to my mind.

When I began to drink green smoothies, I noticed right away that those kinds of cravings disappeared. That was when my husband really noticed the difference in my behavior. In the evening after a hard workday, he would still crave something to eat while I was relaxed and content just reading a book or talking. When Igor saw how happy I was in the evenings, along with the noticeable improvements in my health, he joined me in drinking green smoothies. He started to ask for a cup of "that green stuff" whenever I was making it.

Neither Igor nor I had any illnesses, so in the beginning it was hard to tell if we were just excited or if we really felt better. But soon both Igor and I were able to testify that we experienced rejuvenation, and we began to look younger.

After only two months of drinking smoothies, Igor's mustache and beard started growing blacker, making him look like he did when we first met.

Igor became so enthusiastic about his youthful look that he became the green smoothie champion of my family. He would wake up early and make two or three gallons of smoothie every day: one for me, one for him, and one for Sergei and Valya to share. Both of our children enjoyed including this tasty green drink in their menu and found that they had more energy again. They noticed still more benefits, like the ability to sleep less, more complete eliminations, stronger nails, and most of all, improvement in their teeth, which became less sensitive.

One of my fears was that I would get tired of green smoothies some day and I wouldn't want them any more. But after six months of regular consumption I was enjoying them more than ever. Now I couldn't imagine my life without my green smoothies, as they had become 50 percent of my diet. In addition to smoothies, I ate flax crackers, salads, fruit, and occasionally seeds or nuts. In order to always have the opportunity to make a fresh green smoothie for myself, I purchased an additional Vita-Mix blender for my office. Whenever friends or customers came in, they saw a big green cup next to my computer and I treated them to a sample of my new discovery. To my great satisfaction, everybody loved it, despite their different dietary habits. Unexpectedly, some of my friends and coworkers started to comment on improvements in their health just from the cup of green smoothie they were drinking in my office. No kidding! My Web designer began to crave more raw foods as a result of rather irregular helpings of smoothies and lost fifteen pounds in a couple of months. The woman from the office across the road got rid of her eczema by drinking a cup of green smoothie almost every day. Even the FedEx guy liked it!

Inspired by the warm reception, I wrote an article titled "Ode to Green Smoothie" and e-mailed it to everyone in my Internet address book. Almost instantly I began to receive strong positive feedback and many detailed testimonials from my friends, students, and customers. While I felt compelled to do more research, it looked like the multiple benefits of green smoothies became obvious to everybody who tried them, and the number of people who were drinking green smoothies turned into a "green wave," growing rapidly every day.

5

Why Is It Hard to Love Greens?

Life expectancy would grow by leaps and bounds
if green vegetables smelled as good as bacon.
—DOUG LARSON

Green leaves haven't been included in our food pyramids as a separate group because in modern times it is uncommon to consider greens real food. While carrot tops have several times more nutrients than carrots, the opinion that greens are for rabbits, sheep, and cows has been preventing us from eating carrot tops in our salads. We routinely throw away the most nutritious part of the carrot plant! The roots are more palatable to human taste buds than the tops because the roots contain significantly more sugar and water. The tops are bitter because of the abundance of nutrients in them.

The following charts clearly show the nutritional supremacy of leaves over roots in three different plants: beets, parsley, and turnips.[1] The only three categories in which roots score higher than leaves are in calories, carbohydrates, and sugars (except for turnips). These are the three components that make the roots more palatable to us than the tops. I was impressed with some of these figures. For example, the calcium in beet tops is seven times higher than that of its roots, and vitamin A is 192 times higher in the tops than in the roots. In turnips, vitamin K in the tops is 2,500 (!) times higher than in the roots. The compelling difference between nutrients in these two parts of the plants is clearly indisputable. Think about the thousands of tons of highly nutritious food, the green tops of root vegetables, that are wasted year after year due to our ignorance while the majority of people suffer from chronic nutritional deficiencies.

Naturally, one question comes to mind: Why don't greens taste good to us? Isn't the body wise enough to intuitively crave what it needs? Only a few times in my life have I met people who loved and craved greens. They told me that their parents didn't give them stimulating foods such as candy or fried foods when they were babies. I consider these friends of mine to be the luckiest people in the world. My friend Vanessa becomes ecstatic about a piece of celery or a fresh tomato. Looking at snow peas makes her salivate. Vanessa says,

> Simple food has always tasted best to me. You really cannot appreciate the essence of a food unless you eat it all by itself. Then you can really enjoy its true taste. When my mom and I go to parties, we usually just eat the green leafy garnish from underneath the cuts of cheese. I would prefer it if the kale was on top of the cheese, but at least it's there.

However, most people would be distraught if they came to a party to find only cucumbers, tomatoes, and peas, or even worse, just that bed of greens. It seems clear to me that if we do crave foods with stimulants like sugar, caffeine, and white flour, it means that our intricate bodily homeostasis has become distorted.

In the last few centuries, the human body has changed. The foods that have more stimulating tastes have become more appetizing to us than natural unprocessed foods. Yet everyone recognizes the reality that we cannot thrive on chocolate and pasta alone, no matter how tasty they may be. From my research I have learned that many people would not agree to a bland or bitter diet for the sake of feeling better, even if they had a life-threatening illness. Still, many

Nutritional Comparison of Roots and Greens

BEETS, 100 grams

Nutrients	Beets	Beet Greens
Calories	43.00	22.00
Protein (g)	1.61	2.20
Fat Total (g)	0.17	0.13
Carbohydrate (g)	9.56	4.33
Fiber – Total (g)	2.80	3.70
Sugar – Total (g)	6.76	.50
Calcium (mg)	16.00	117.00
Iron (mg)	0.80	2.57
Magnesium (mg)	23.00	70.00
Phosphorus (mg)	40.00	41.00
Potassium (mg)	325.00	762.00
Sodium (mg)	78.00	226.00
Zinc (mg)	0.35	0.38
Copper (mg)	0.08	0.19
Manganese (mg)	0.33	0.39
Selenium (mg)	0.70	0.90
Vitamin C (mg)	4.90	30.00
Thiamin (mg)	0.03	0.10
Riboflavin (mg)	0.04	0.22
Niacin (mg)	0.33	0.40
Vitamin B6 (mg)	0.07	0.11
Folate – Total (mcg)	109.00	15.00
Food – Folate (mcg)	109.00	15.00
Folate – DFE (mcg_DEF)	109.00	15.00
Vitamin B12 (mcg)	0.00	0.00
Vitamin A (IU)	33.00	6,326.00
Retinol (mcg)	0.00	0.00
Vitamin E (mg)	0.04	1.50
Vitamin K (mcg)	0.20	400.00
Fat – Saturated (g)	0.03	0.02
Fat – Monosaturated (g)	0.03	0.03
Fat – Polysaturated (g)	0.06	0.05
Cholesterol (mg)	0.0	0.00

Nutritional Comparison of Roots and Greens

PARSLEY, 100 grams

Nutrients	Parsnips (root)	Parsley
Calories	75.00	36.00
Protein (g)	1.20	2.97
Fat Total (g)	0.30	0.79
Carbohydrate (g)	17.99	6.33
Fiber – Total (g)	4.90	3.30
Sugar – Total (g)	4.80	.85
Calcium (mg)	36.00	138.00
Iron (mg)	0.59	6.20
Magnesium (mg)	29.00	50.00
Phosphorus (mg)	71.00	58.00
Potassium (mg)	375.00	554.00
Sodium (mg)	10.00	56.00
Zinc (mg)	0.59	1.07
Copper (mg)	0.12	0.15
Manganese (mg)	0.56	0.16
Selenium (mg)	1.80	0.10
Vitamin C (mg)	17.00	133.00
Thiamin (mg)	0.09	0.09
Riboflavin (mg)	0.05	0.10
Niacin (mg)	0.70	1.31
Vitamin B6 (mg)	0.09	0.09
Folate – Total (mcg)	67.00	152.00
Food – Folate (mcg)	67.00	152.00
Folate – DFE (mcg_DEF)	67.00	152.00
Vitamin B12 (mcg)	0.00	0.00
Vitamin A (IU)	0.00	8,424.00
Retinol (mcg)	0.00	0.00
Vitamin E (mg)	1.49	0.75
Vitamin K (mcg)	22.50	1,640.00
Fat – Saturated (g)	0.05	0.13
Fat – Monosaturated (g)	0.11	0.29
Fat – Polysaturated (g)	0.05	0.12
Cholesterol (mg)	0.0	0.0

Nutritional Comparison of Roots and Greens

TURNIPS, 100 grams

Nutrients	Turnips	Turnip Greens
Calories	28.00	32.00
Protein (g)	0.90	1.50
Fat Total (g)	0.10	0.30
Carbohydrate (g)	6.43	7.13
Fiber – Total (g)	1.80	3.20
Sugar – Total (g)	3.80	0.81
Calcium (mg)	30.00	190.00
Iron (mg)	0.30	1.10
Magnesium (mg)	11.00	31.00
Phosphorus (mg)	27.00	42.00
Potassium (mg)	191.00	296.00
Sodium (mg)	67.00	40.00
Zinc (mg)	0.27	0.19
Copper (mg)	0.09	0.35
Manganese (mg)	0.13	0.47
Selenium (mg)	0.70	1.20
Vitamin C (mg)	21.00	60.00
Thiamin (mg)	0.04	0.07
Riboflavin (mg)	0.03	0.10
Niacin (mg)	0.40	0.60
Vitamin B6 (mg)	0.09	0.26
Folate – Total (mcg)	15.00	194.00
Food – Folate (mcg)	15.00	194.00
Folate – DFE (mcg_DEF)	15.00	194.00
Vitamin B12 (mcg)	0.00	0.00
Vitamin A (IU)	0.00	0.00
Retinol (mcg)	0.00	0.00
Vitamin E (mg)	0.03	2.86
Vitamin K (mcg)	0.10	251.00
Fat – Saturated (g)	0.01	0.07
Fat – Monosaturated (g)	0.01	0.02
Fat – Polysaturated (g)	0.05	0.12
Cholesterol (mg)	0.00	0.00

are continuing to ask, "What are we supposed to eat? How are we supposed to feed our children in order to achieve better health?" Remarkably, green smoothies are not only nutritious but also delightfully palatable, even to children.

I strongly believe that it is possible to restore our ability to like and crave healthy foods. We can learn to live on a natural, healthy diet even though we have developed some powerful, unnatural cravings. Over time my smoothies changed in color, going from a light green to a dark emerald as my cravings for a much greener blend increased. I began putting 70 to 80 percent greens in my blender and only a handful of fruit—for example, one bunch of dandelions and two tomatoes. I named this concoction my "super green smoothie." I urge you to start with really sweet and delicious green smoothies and progress to darker smoothies only if you enjoy them. I believe that eating plenty of ripe organic fruit is also necessary for vibrant health. The presence of high-quality greens in one's diet has proven to encourage healthier food cravings, as you may see from the testimonials at the end of this book.

6

———————

Greens: A New Food Group

I wonder how greens such as kale, romaine lettuce, spinach, and carrot tops got classified as vegetables. Why do we call foods from completely different food groups "vegetables" when they look different and contain different sets of nutrients? A produce manager from a local health-food store complained to me that his customers often got confused when looking for a particular ingredient among the 150-plus types of produce all gathered under the single name "vegetables." This man had worked in the produce section for more than ten years. He suggested that the produce be divided into several different groups of plant foods with specific characteristics, for example, roots (carrots, beets, daikon, etc.), flowers (broccoli, cauliflower, artichokes, etc.), and nonsweet fruit (cucumbers, zucchini, squash, tomatoes, etc.). Combining foods with similar nutritional values would not only help shoppers find necessary ingredients faster but would also help them become familiar with more plant foods and increase the variety of vegetarian foods in their diet.

Obviously, plants are not considered important enough to be classified properly. Even at a regular supermarket, one can see that other food departments have more detailed classifications. For example, the meat department is divided into poultry, fish, and red meat, which in turn is subdivided into smaller sections such as veal, ground meats, bones, and byproducts. Every item is carefully categorized, specifying which part of the animal it is from. Cheeses have their own specifications. Nobody would ever classify cheese and meat together in one "sandwich food" group because it would be inconvenient and unclear. Yet this kind of confusion and error continually occurs in the produce section. Some of these errors are quite serious, to such a degree that they could cause health problems. For example, placing starchy roots in the same category with tomatoes and rhubarb could prompt customers to make improper food-combining choices. Many nutritionists believe in the importance of proper food combining,[1] and have found that starchy tubers combined in one meal with sour fruits or vegetables can create fermentation and gas in our intestines.

Placing greens in the same category as vegetables has caused people to mistakenly apply the combining rules for starchy vegetables to greens. Driven by this confusion, many concerned people have written to me inquiring if blending fruits with greens was proper food combining. They had heard that "fruits and vegetables did not mix well." Yes, to combine starchy vegetables with fruits is not a good idea; such a combination can cause gas in the intestines. However, *greens are not vegetables* and greens are not starchy. In fact, greens are the only food group that helps digest other foods through stimulating the secretion of digestive enzymes. Thus greens can be combined with any other foods. It has been recorded that chimpanzees often consume fruits and leaves from the same tree at the same feeding time. In fact, Jane Goodall and other researchers have observed them rolling fruits inside of leaves and eating them as "sandwiches."

There is yet another great misconception that results from placing greens and vegetables in the same category. Such inappropriate generalizations have lead researchers to the erroneous conclusion that greens are a poor source of protein. Contrary to this popular belief, greens are an excellent source of protein, as you will see in the following chapter.

I propose that we separate greens from vegetables, now and forevermore. Greens have never received proper attention and have never been researched adequately because they have been incorrectly identified as vegetables. We don't even have a proper name for greens in most languages. The name "dark green leafy vegetables" is long and inconvenient to use, similar to "the animal with horns that gives milk."

We don't have complete nutritional data about greens. For this book I had to collect bits and pieces of information out of books and magazines from different countries, and I still don't have all the data. I have not, for example, been able to find the complete nutritional content of carrot tops anywhere. Nevertheless, I have found enough to draw some essential conclusions: *greens are the primary food group that matches human nutritional needs most completely.*

The following chart is a list of all essential minerals and vitamins that are recommended by the U.S. Department of Agriculture (USDA) and a list of these nutrients available in kale and lambsquarters (an edible weed). Based on this data, we can conclude that greens are the most essential food for humans.

Often people ask me what quantity of smoothies they should drink every day. I recommend that they consume one to two quarts (liters) of green smoothies per day in addition to their existing diet. Typically people begin to notice a beneficial effect on their health within one or two days. To appreciate the value of green smoothies, I challenge you to find another food that is as nutritious in so many aspects as a green smoothie. Green smoothies are very tasty and easy to prepare as well.

Essential Mineral and Vitamin Content

LAMBSQUARTERS (a weed) and KALE

Nutrients Adequate Intake or RDA16	Kale One pound raw	Lambsquarters (weed) One pound raw
Folic Acid – 400 mcg/day	132 mcg	136.0 mcg
Niacin – 16 mg/day	4.8 mg	5.4 mg
Pantothenic Acid – 5 mg/day	0.68 mg	0.45 mg
Riboflavin (B2) – 1.3 mg/day	0.68 mg	0.9 mg
Thiamin (B1) – 1.2 mg/day	0.68 mg	1.8 mg
Vitamin A – 900 mcg/day	21,012.0 mcg	15,800.0 mcg
Vitamin B6 – 1.3 mg/day	68.0 mg	8.0 mg
Vitamin B12 – 2.4 mcg/day	data unavailable	data unavailable
Vitamin C – 90 mg/day	547.0 mg	363.0 mg
Vitamin D – 5 mcg/day (based on absence of adequate exposure to sunlight)*	data unavailable see note	data unavailable see note
Vitamin E – 15 mg/day	data unavailable	data unavailable
Vitamin K – 120 mcg/day	3,720.0 mcg	data unavailable

Minerals

Calcium – 1,000 mg/day	615.0 mg	1,403.0 mg
Iron – 10 mg/day	7.5 mg	5.4 mg
Magnesium – 400 mg/day	155.0 mg	154.0 mg
Phosphorus – 700 mg/day	255.0 mg	327.0 mg
Potassium – 4.7 g/day	2.1 g	2.1 g
Sodium – 1.5 g/day	0.2 g	0.2 g
Zinc – 15 mg/day	2.0 mg	1.8 mg
Copper – 1.5 mg/day	1.4 mg	1.4 mg
Manganese – 10 mg/day	3.4 mg	3.6 mg
Selenium – 70 mcg/day	4.0 mcg	4.1 mc

*For a Caucasian with medium skin pigmentation, exposure of the face, hands, and arms for five minutes two or three times a week for three-fourths of the year actually eliminates the need for dietary intake of vitamin D.

To demonstrate how nutritious green smoothies are, I have created a comprehensive nutritional analysis for three green smoothies using recipes from this book. The complete analysis of these smoothies is very detailed and lengthy. Below are short versions of these charts, showing the nutritional content of one quart (or one liter) of three different green smoothies. To view a complete version of the nutritional analysis of these three smoothies, please use the following links:

Summer Delight
http://nutritiondata.self.com/facts/recipe/1702214/2

Strawberry Field
http://nutritiondata.self.com/facts/recipe/1702245/2

Sweet and Sour
http://nutritiondata.self.com/facts/recipe/1702272/2

I invite you to take advantage of the valuable and helpful Web site http://nutritiondata.self.com, where you may calculate your own recipes' nutritional content using the latest and most accurate data that comes directly from the USDA's National Nutrient Database.

Summer Delight Smoothie

Peaches, 2 cups, sliced (308g)
Spinach, raw, 5 cups (150g)
Water, 2 cups, 16 fl oz (237g)
Preparation: Blend well

Nutrition Facts

Serving size 932g (1 liter)

Amount Per Serving

Calories	155	Calories from Fat	11

% Daily Value*

Total Fat 1g	2%
Saturated Fat 0g	
Trans Fat 0g	
Cholesterol 0mg	
Sodium 123mg	5%
Total Carbohydrate 36g	12%
Dietary Fiber 8g	32%
Sugars 29g	
Protein 7g	

Vitamin A	301%	†Vitamin C	104%
Calcium	17%	†Iron	27%

*Percent Daily Values are based on a 2,000-calorie diet.
Your daily values may be higher or lower depending on
your calorie needs.

NutritionData.com

Strawberry Field Smoothie

Banana, 1 cup, sliced (150g)
Lettuce, Cos or Romaine, 5 cups, shredded (235g)
Strawberries, 1 cup, halved (152g)
Water, 2 cups, 16 fl oz (237g)
Preparation: Blend well

Nutrition Facts

Serving size 1,000g (1 liter)

Amount Per Serving

Calories 222 Calories from Fat 14

% **Daily Value***

Total Fat 2g	3%
Saturated Fat 0g	
Trans Fat 0g	
Cholesterol 0mg	
Sodium 27mg	1%
Total Carbohydrate 54g	18%
Dietary Fiber 12g	48%
Sugars 29g	

Protein 6g

Vitamin A	41.2%	†Vitamin C	65%
Calcium	11%	†Iron	19%

*Percent Daily Values are based on a 2,000-calorie diet.
Your daily values may be higher or lower depending on
your calorie needs.

NutritionData.com

Sweet and Sour Smoothie

Apricots, 4 (35g)
Banana, 1 large (136g)
Blueberries, 2 ounces (28g)
Lettuce, red leaf, 200 grams
Water, 2 cups, 16 fl oz (237g)
Preparation: Blend well

Nutrition Facts

Serving size 1,000g (1 liter)

Amount Per Serving

Calories	252	Calories from Fat	14

% Daily Value*

Total Fat 2g	2%
Saturated Fat 0g	
Trans Fat 0g	
Cholesterol 0mg	
Sodium 63mg	3%
Total Carbohydrate 59g	20%
Dietary Fiber 9g	38%
Sugars 36g	
Protein 7g	

Vitamin A	356%	†Vitamin C	64%
Calcium	14%	†Iron	19%

*Percent Daily Values are based on a 2,000-calorie diet. Your daily values may be higher or lower depending on your calorie needs.

NutritionData.com

7

The Abundance of Proteins in Greens

*I submit that scientists have not yet explored the hidden
possibilities of the innumerable seeds, leaves, and fruits
for giving the fullest possible nutrition to mankind.*
—MAHATMA GANDHI

Every protein molecule consists of a chain of amino acids. An essential amino acid is one that cannot be synthesized by the body and therefore must be supplied as part of the diet. Humans must include adequate amounts of nine amino acids in their diet.

Professor T. Colin Campbell shows in his book *The China Study* that the U.S. Recommended Dietary Allowance (RDA) for protein is greatly overestimated. Studies of the diets of chimpanzees compared to that of humans confirm the same truth. "Chimpanzees maintain a fairly low and constant protein intake, due to their focus on fruit ..."[1]

I have looked at the nutritional content of dozens of green vegetables and I was pleased to see that the amino acids that were low in one plant were high in another. In other words, if we maintain a variety of greens in our diet, we will cover all essential amino acids in abundance.

Look at the chart of the essential amino acid content in kale and lambsquarters on the next page. I have chosen kale because it is available in most produce markets. Lambsquarters is one of the most common edible weeds that grows in various climates. Most farmers should be able to identify lambsquarters for you.

In the left-hand column you can see the recommended amounts of essential amino acids for an average adult.[2] In the right column are the amounts of those amino acids contained in lambsquarters and kale. Notice that dark-green leafy vegetables contain similar or greater amounts of amino acids than the RDA.

As you can see from this chart, one pound of kale has even more protein than the USDA's recommended daily serving. But by erroneously placing all parts of plants (roots, stalks, blossoms, spears, greens, etc.) into the category of vegetables and assuming they have the same properties, we have mistakenly concluded that greens are a poor source of protein. This inaccurate conclusion has led to malnourishment and suffering for decades. The lack of research on the nutritional content of greens has led to great confusion among the majority of people, including many professionals. As Dr. Joel Fuhrman writes in his book *Eat to Live,* "Even physicians and dietitians ... are surprised to learn that ... when you eat large quantities of green vegetables, you receive a considerable amount of protein."[3] In her lectures, author and teacher Tonya Zavasta shares a clever observation: It is a known fact that milk is rich in protein, but, she says, we never question how the milk becomes full of protein. Do cows produce such large quantities of protein daily out of thin air? In Russia, dairy farmers often brag about the quality of their milk by saying, "This milk is so fresh that only four hours ago it was still grass!"

Whether by phone, e-mail, or at a lecture, every day I am asked the question: "Where do I get my protein?" Being aware of the confusion around vegetables, I understand why this question has become so common. Since most people are not aware that greens have an

Essential Amino Acid Content

LAMBSQUARTERS (a weed) and KALE

Amino Acids	RDA for average adult (mg/day)	Content (mg) Lambsquarters One pound raw
Histidine	560	527
Isoleucine	70	1,149
Leucine	980	1,589
Lysine	840	1,607
Methionine + cystine	910	222 + 404 = 626
Phenylalanine + tyrosine	980	754 + 795 = 1,549
Threonine	490	740
Tryptophan	245	173
Valine	700	1,026

Amino Acids	RDA for average adult (mg/day)	Content (mg) in KALE One pound raw
Histidine	560	313
Isoleucine	70	895
Leucine	980	1,051
Lysine	840	895
Methionine + cystine	910	145 + 200 = 345
Phenylalanine + tyrosine	980	766 + 532 = 1,298
Threonine	490	668
Tryptophan	245	182
Valine	700	820

abundance of readily available essential amino acids, they try to consume protein from other food groups known for their rich protein content. However, let me explain the difference between the complex proteins found in meat, dairy, and fish, and the individual amino acids found in fruits, vegetables, and especially in greens.

It is clear that the body has to work a lot less when creating protein from the assortment of individual amino acids from greens rather than from the already-combined long molecules of protein that are assembled according to the foreign pattern of a totally different creature such as a cow or a chicken. I would like to explain the difference between complex proteins and individual amino acids with a simple anecdote.

Imagine that you have to make a wedding dress for your daughter. Consuming the complex proteins that we get from cows or other creatures is like going to the secondhand store and buying many other people's used dresses, coming home, and spending several hours ripping apart pieces of the dresses that you like and combining them into a new wedding dress for your daughter. This alternative would take a lot of time and energy and leave a great deal of garbage. You could never make a perfect dress this way.

Consuming individual amino acids is like taking your daughter to a fabric store to buy beautiful new fabric, lace, buttons, ribbons, threads, and pearls. With these essential elements you can make a beautiful dress that fits her unique body perfectly. Similarly, when you eat greens, you "purchase" new amino acids, freshly made by sunshine and chlorophyll, that the body will use to rebuild its parts according to your own unique DNA.

Contrary to this, your body would have a hard time trying to make a perfect molecule of protein out of someone else's molecules, which consist of totally different combinations of amino acids. Plus your body would most likely receive a lot of unnecessary pieces that are hard to digest. These pieces would be floating around in your blood like garbage for a long time, causing allergies and other health problems. Professor W. A. Walker from the Department of Nutrition at the Harvard School of Public Health states that "Incompletely digested protein fragments may be absorbed into the bloodstream. The absorption of these large molecules contributes to the development of food allergies and immunological disorders."[4]

The ironic result of consuming this imperfect source of protein, animal protein, is that many people develop deficiencies in essential amino acids. Such deficiencies are not only dangerous to our health but also dramatically change our perception of life and the way we feel and behave. In producing neurotransmitters, the body uses essential amino acids such as tyrosine, tryptophan, glutamine, and histidine. Neurotransmitters are the natural chemicals that facilitate communication between brain cells. These substances govern our emotions, memory, moods, behavior, learning abilities, and sleep patterns. For the last three decades, neurotransmitters have been the focus of mental health research.

According to the research of Julia Ross, a specialist in nutritional psychology,[5] if your body lacks certain amino acids, you may develop strong symptoms of mental and physiological imbalance and severe cravings for unwanted substances.

For example, let us consider tyrosine and phenylalanine. The symptoms of a deficiency in these amino acids can cause:

- depression
- lack of focus and concentration
- lack of energy
- attention deficit disorder

In addition, the symptoms of a deficiency in these amino acids may lead to cravings for:

- sweets
- aspartame
- caffeine
- starch

- alcohol
- cocaine
- chocolate
- marijuana
- tobacco

Using available data from official sources[6] I have calculated the amounts of these two essential amino acids that we can receive from either chicken or dark-green endive:

Chicken (one serving):
222 mg tyrosine
261 mg phenylalanine

Endive (one head):
205 mg tyrosine
272 mg phenylalanine

As you can see, contrary to popular opinion, there are plenty of high-quality protein building blocks in greens. According to Professor T. Colin Campbell, "There is a mountain of compelling evidence showing that so-called 'low-quality' plant protein, which allows for slow but steady synthesis of new proteins, is the healthiest type of protein."[7] For example, the protein from greens doesn't have cancer as a side effect. Yet in many books, greens are not even listed as a protein source because greens have not been researched enough.

Greens provide sufficient protein to build muscle in grazing animals. I received this testimony from my very first American friend, a farmer with a BA in psychology from Harvard University, Peter Hagerty of Maine:

When our sheep are in the barn eating *concentrated feed* such as ground corn and oats, they gain weight much more *quickly,* but young lambs, once they reach 120 lbs or 90% of slaughter weight, begin putting this concentrated food into *fat* rather than muscle which is not advantageous for the consumer who has to trim this fat off and throw it away. If the lambs are *grass fed,* they grow more *slowly* but they can reach full slaughter weight with *very little fat.* So my observations are: concentrates seem to put on easily burnable fats and grasses put on quality muscle.

In summary, greens provide protein in the form of individual amino acids. These amino acids are easier for the body to utilize than complex proteins. A variety of greens can supply all the protein we need to sustain each of our unique bodies.

8

Fiber: The Magic Sponge

Dr. Bernard Jensen, DC, PhD, one of the most renowned nutrition experts in the world and author of many popular health books, stated that:

> Any cleansing program should begin in the colon. ... In the 50 years I've spent helping people to overcome illness, disability, and disease, it has become crystal clear that poor bowel management lies at the root of most people's health problems. In treating over 300,000 patients, it is the bowel that invariably has to be cared for first before any effective healing can take place.[1]

The main purpose of consuming fiber is elimination. Without fiber, complete elimination is nearly impossible, if it is possible at all. The human body is miraculously built in such a way that almost all the toxins from every part of the body, including millions of dead cells, end up daily in the human sewage system—the colon. The colon fills up with waste matter so full of poison that we look at it with disgust, not daring to touch it. In order to eliminate this matter, the body needs fiber.

There are two main kinds of fiber: soluble and insoluble. Soluble fiber, found in fruit, beans, peas, oat bran, and especially in chia seeds, has a gel-like consistency that improves bowel movements by increasing the volume of bulk in the colon. Soluble fiber binds together cholesterol in the small intestines and takes it out of the body. Certain kinds of soluble fiber, such as pectin (found in apples) and guar gums (found in chia seeds, oatmeal, legumes, and mangoes), slow down the release of the sugars contained in the foods we eat, thus reducing the risk of diabetes.

Insoluble fiber is found primarily in greens, peels, nuts, seeds, beans, and the husks of grains. The elimination system is very complex; it has been perfected by nature in every minute action. I'll try to explain this complicated process with a very simple example. Under a microscope, insoluble fiber looks like a sponge, and indeed it serves us as a miraculous sponge because every piece of it can absorb many times more toxins than its own volume. Have you ever wondered why people like to have a sponge in the kitchen? We never use something smooth, like paper or plastic, to wipe dirty counters clean. Sponges are fibrous, and they make the job of cleaning easier by absorbing dirt. So does insoluble fiber: it grabs the toxins and takes them out of the body and into the toilet. Insoluble fiber is much better than any sponge because it can hold several times more toxins than its own size. I call it a magic sponge.

If we do not consume fiber, most of the toxic waste accumulates in our body. Our body is constructed in such a marvelous way that all the toxins are directed to the bowels. This is the human body's sewage system. We need to understand that we have to eliminate many pounds of toxins regularly.

Where do toxins come from? They come from inhaling dust and asbestos, from undigested food, ingested heavy metals, and from pesticides. But a large amount of toxins also come from the dead cells of our own bodies. Because we know that cells are tiny, we tend to think that the cell could not add much to the amount of waste in our body. However, let's keep in mind that every year as much as 98 percent of the total number of atoms in our body are replaced.[2] That means anywhere from seventy to one hundred pounds of dead cells, or more, should be passing out of our system each year. If they don't, the dead cells of our own body can be one of the most toxic kinds of waste because they begin to rot right away. It is important to understand that when we do not consume enough fiber, we accumulate a lot more waste than our bodies can handle.

Just as one cannot clean a kitchen without a sponge, the human body cannot eliminate without fiber. Picture yourself being challenged to clean some large dirty space like a garage with nothing but plastic wrap. I would give up. The human body won't give up, but if there is no fiber, the first thing that happens is that our skin tries to take on the elimination "job" and as a result becomes rough and bumpy. When our bowels are clogged, our body attempts to excrete more mucus through our eyes, nose, and throat, and we sweat a lot more—the body uses every possible channel to eliminate, but it's like pushing the garbage out through a window screen instead of the door. By consuming enough insoluble fiber, we unlock the door to eliminate toxins from the body the easy and normal way.

Now, you are probably wondering how much fiber we need to consume for optimal health benefits. According to research, the average wild chimpanzee consumes over two hundred grams of fiber per day.[3] When I read that, I calculated how much fiber I consumed each day. I came up with only three grams because I consumed a lot of my vegetables in the form of juice. Very often I would juice my fruits and vegetables rather than "waste" my time and effort on chewing them. About thirty years ago, in the first books I read about juicing, I learned that fiber was not digestible, contained no nutrients, and served merely as a strain on the human intestinal tract. After that, juicing became one of my regular habits. I was proudly juicing for days, even weeks, trying to "cleanse" myself of toxins, and I considered myself to be maintaining a very healthy diet. So I was astounded by the comparison of the chimpanzee's two hundred grams of fiber with my own three. Moreover, I realized how harmful it was for my health when I consumed zero fiber by juicing all the time. I decided that I couldn't afford to throw my fiber in the compost anymore. While green smoothies are definitely superior to juices, however, I recognize that in a number of circumstances juices may be preferable to smoothies, as in the case of people with irritable bowel syndrome and other conditions.

Albert Mosséri, the famous French doctor of natural hygiene, has radically changed the classical Sheltonian method of fasting on water. After supervising four thousand long-term water fasts conducted at his clinic, he came to the extraordinary conclusion that long-term fasts were a "risky waste of time." He now oversees much shorter water fasts followed by what he calls "half-fasts," in which he introduces a limited amount of food rich in fiber in addition to water. During this important stage of healing, his patients receive only one pound of fruits and one pound of vegetables daily until their elimination is complete.[4] Dr. Mosséri states that switching to this half-fast method has accelerated elimination to such a degree that one hundred percent of his patients develop profound signs of a deep cleansing process in the form of a dark coating on their tongues, often charcoal black or dark brown.

Enormous amounts of research on dietary fiber have been done all around the world since the beginning of the last century. We now have undeniable evidence of fiber's many healing properties. Here are some of them:

- Fiber can strengthen a diseased heart.[5]
- Fiber reduces cholesterol, which decreases the risk of heart disease.
- Fiber prevents many different kinds of cancer, reduces cancer risks, and binds carcinogens.
- Fiber can lessen the risk of diabetes and improve already-diagnosed diabetes.
- Fiber steadies blood sugar levels by slowing down the absorption of sugar.[6]
- Fiber can strengthen the immune system.
- Fiber keeps our bowels healthy, relieves constipation, and promotes regularity.
- Fiber prevents gallstones.[7]
- Fiber promotes healthy intestinal bacteria.
- Fiber helps us lose weight and curbs overeating.
- Fiber binds up excess estrogen.
- Fiber prevents ulcers.

The U.S. Recommended Daily Allowance for fiber is thirty grams per day. The average American consumes between ten and fifteen grams of fiber per day.[8] That is far from sufficient. Considering the fact that these ten tiny grams of fiber would have to absorb and move out several huge pounds of waste matter, ten grams is almost nothing. I think insufficient fiber intake is one of the main reasons for premature aging in humans. Look at any animal that lives in the wild. One can hardly guess the age of a deer, zebra, eagle, or giraffe. Whether they are at the age of two or fifteen years old, they look relatively the same. Wild animals only begin to slow down during the last weeks before they die. On the other hand, it is often easy to guess the age of humans within five years. But I have also seen many people start to look younger once they improved their elimination.

I believe we should consume thirty to fifty grams of fiber per day or more. However, we have to increase the intake of fiber gradually. It can be dangerous to switch overnight from ten grams to fifty.

Many of our bodies have degenerated over the decades due to the consumption of processed foods. In addition, we have adopted many unnatural practices such as exercising too little and spending most of the time indoors. Therefore, we need to reintroduce healthy habits into our lives slowly to give our bodies time to readjust. Green smoothies are perfect for this gradual shift. Other sources of fiber, and especially fiber in pill form, can often create too drastic an increase of fiber in the diet too quickly, which can result in a bloated feeling and increased gas. Such unpleasant side effects can cause people to give up before they even get a chance to experience the health benefits of fiber.

Fiber is an important component in the diet of chimpanzees. As I noted, they consume two hundred grams of fiber per day. In addition to eating many fiber-rich fruits and leaves, they supplement their diet with pith and bark, both of which consist of approximately 44 percent fiber.

Flaxseed is a perfect addition to the human diet. It is very high in both soluble and insoluble fiber. It contains 26 percent fiber (14 percent soluble, 12 percent insoluble). Just one-eighth of a cup, or two tablespoons, of flaxseed contains six grams of fiber.

I recommend adding flaxseed to your diet regularly. Flaxseeds have a tough outer coating and should be freshly ground to release the most nutritional benefit. You can grind whole seeds with a coffee grinder or in a Vita-Mix dry container. I recommend adding one or two tablespoons of ground flax meal to your salads, soups, and other dishes. Flaxseed is also a good source of omega-3 fatty acids and it is by far nature's richest source of plant lignin, an important anticancer phytonutrient. My family has been intuitively adding flaxseed to our meals every day, either in the form of crackers or as flax meal.

While chimpanzees consume a lot of fiber, they spend several hours every day chewing their foods. In our busy modern life, we are used to consuming meals in short periods of time. Due to our rushed lifestyle, our food has generally become too soft, such as mashed potatoes, bread, or rice. Our jaws, like any bone, require resistance in order to maintain healthy bone density. I have even developed my own jaw exerciser, which I chew one to two minutes daily to compensate for my lack of chewing firm foods. If you are interested, you may view this product at my Web site, http://jaw exerciser.com.

Green smoothies take only three to five minutes to prepare, including cleanup. One quart or liter of green smoothie contains approximately twelve to eighteen grams of fiber, depending on the water content and the type of fruit used.

If you consume dairy, meat, poultry, or other animal products, you might want to know that all animal foods contain zero fiber. In order to eliminate well, one needs to consume plant foods. The more plant foods we consume, the more fiber we get. I would like to give you an idea how many fruits, greens, and veggies to consume. One medium-size apple contains three grams of fiber, as does a banana or a mango. A handful of kale or chard contains one gram. While juices are probably the most nourishing food there is, blended smoothies are both nourishing and cleansing. Since deficiency and toxicity are the main causes of diseases, it is best if we both nourish and cleanse our bodies. For the sake of fiber and elimination, drink your smoothies regularly.

9

Greens for Homeostasis

Look at this body! It's a work of art. No improvements
can be made ... divinely put together.
—DR. BERNARD JENSEN[1]

The main difference between living things and non-living things is that living entities can repair themselves and thus to a great extent can adapt to changes in their environment, while things that are not alive can be broken and destroyed. For example, if you tear a leaf off a plant, the plant can grow a new leaf. If you cut the skin on your finger, your skin will heal itself. Alternately, nonliving things like rocks or artificial constructions, no matter how big and strong, cannot repair themselves if damaged. For instance, after catastrophes such as earthquakes, avalanches, and tornadoes, people have to rebuild their homes, roads, power plants, and so on.

This extraordinary ability of all living organisms to repair themselves is the only power that can heal any illness. All other healing techniques invented by people can be successful only if they are directed toward helping the body's own natural ability to regulate itself. A human body can heal a disease only when all bodily substances, such as lymph, blood, hormones, and countless others, are maintained within optimal parameters.

The physiological process that keeps all substances in the body at the levels necessary for optimal body health is called homeostasis.[2] This process is extremely complex, and a complete understanding of its mechanisms goes far beyond our three-dimensional imagination. Homeostasis is the most important process in the body, and if we are helping our homeostasis, we are taking the best possible care of our health.

How can we take care of our homeostasis when it is out of our reach? The process of homeostasis in the human body is tightly connected to the endocrine system. Homeostatic balance depends on the performance of the endocrine glands. If the glands do not secrete the proper amount of hormones, the homeostatic balance in the body will shift, and disease could start.

The glands of the endocrine system and the hormones they release influence almost every cell, organ, and function of our body. The endocrine system is instrumental in regulating mood, growth and development, tissue function, and metabolism as well as sexual function and reproductive processes.

To make it really simple, the endocrine system in a human body acts like a highly efficient superfactory that manufactures and supplies every substance requested by any gland or organ at any time in the precise quantity required. What does such a factory need? An abundance of high-quality supplies. Similarly, the endocrine system in our body absolutely needs all nutrients, including vitamins, amino acids, carbohydrates, essential fatty acids, minerals, and all trace elements. Supplying all of these nutrients to our body is critical for good health.

Greens match all of these purposes better than any other food, and when blended, the nutrients from greens are absorbed more efficiently and provide many times more nutrients than other foods, including traditionally made salads. In other words, by drinking green smoothies we support our homeostatic balance in the most optimal way.

I wish I had known this information ten years ago when my mother was still alive. She was only sixty-six, a beautiful, adventurous woman, when she was diagnosed with cancer one year after she swam in a river near Chernobyl. I could have explained to her now very clearly how the body can heal. I am sure that Mom would have refused chemotherapy because those poisonous chemicals ruined her already weakened homeostasis. I would have nourished her to health instead. I understand now that supporting, not destroying, homeostasis is what gives a body the greatest chance to heal. She might still be with us.

I have met many people who have survived cancers much more severe than what my mother had by incorporating more greens into their diet. The human body is so wonderfully made that it can even reproduce perfect new human beings. How dare we doubt that the body can heal itself? When we understand the mechanism of homeostasis, it becomes clear that through this unique natural system, the human body can heal not only a cold or recover from injury but heal any disease, even cancer. The only assistance we can offer is to provide sufficient nourishment and elimination. Fortunately, green smoothies can provide such help.

10

The Significance of Stomach Acid

How many people know what their concentration of stomach acid is? How many of us appreciate its importance for our overall health? Almost nobody recognizes how crucial it is to have normal levels of hydrochloric acid in the stomach. I don't know why none of the many doctors I have visited over the years have ever asked me about my hydrochloric acid or tested it for me. I've never heard my friends talk about their stomach acid. I was grateful to learn about its importance from a veterinarian who was helping me create a healthy diet for my dog.

To my surprise, I found scores of books and scientific articles about the connection between the level of hydrochloric acid and human health. This topic has been studied for decades. Professor W. A. Walker from the Department of Nutrition at the Harvard School of Public Health states that "Medical researchers since the 1930s have been concerned about the consequences of hypochlorhydria. While all the health consequences are still not entirely clear, some have been well documented."[1]

Low stomach acidity (hypochlorhydria) is a condition that occurs when the human body is unable to produce adequate quantities of stomach acid. Low stomach acidity inevitably and dramatically impacts digestion and absorption of most nutrients necessary for health. Most minerals, including such important ones as iron, zinc, calcium, and the B-complex vitamins (folic acid and others) need certain amounts of stomach acids in order to be absorbed at all. Without stomach acid, nutritional deficiencies inevitably develop and lead to disease.

Besides absorption, stomach acid has many other important functions. For instance, stomach acid is supposed to destroy all harmful microorganisms, pathogenic bacteria, parasites and their eggs, and fungi that enter the body through the mouth. Therefore, if stomach acid is insufficient, there is no barrier against parasites. I have spoken with a gastroenterologist who takes test samples of stomach acid from his patients and often finds several kinds of parasites flourishing in the very place where they are supposed to be killed. I want my stomach acid to be strong for this reason alone.

Stomach acid helps to digest large protein molecules.[2] If stomach acid is low, incompletely digested protein fragments get absorbed into the bloodstream and cause allergies and immunological disorders.

The natural level of hydrochloric acid (HCl) decreases as we age, especially after the age of forty, which is when most people begin to develop gray hair as a result of nutritional deficiencies caused by lowered stomach acid. I have observed that most people diagnosed with very low stomach acid have noticeably more gray hair. There are numerous well-documented accounts of people's natural hair color returning as a result of consuming blended greens on a regular basis, Ann Wigmore being one of them.

Hydrochloric acid can also start decreasing early in life if we abuse our gastrointestinal tract, or our entire body, through food excesses, chemical use, and stress. Overeating, especially overconsumption of fats and proteins, wears out the parietal cells of the stomach that secrete HCl.[3]

Indigenous peoples throughout history have had many different types of diets, depending on their environment. What they had in common, however, was that they all ate large amounts of fiber. Researchers have estimated that *Australopithecus* and some other indigenous peoples consumed roughly 150 grams of fiber daily.[4] Looking at this number, it's easy to infer that the acidity of their stomachs was quite strong—a lot stronger than ours. They also had much stronger teeth, jaws, and jaw muscles. They were able to chew this rough stringy food to a creamy consistency in their mouths, and then their stomachs continued digesting this well-chewed matter by applying hydrochloric acid. Our bodies have dramatically changed since then. Do an experiment: take a piece of any vegetable or green leaf, sit down, and chew it as long as you can. Just before you are ready to swallow it, spit it out onto your palm and take a look at it. You will see that it will still be far from a creamy consistency. Keep in mind that your body would only be able to assimilate nutrients from the tiniest particles. Large particles won't get digested and will turn into acidic waste. A friend of mine who is a doctor, and frequently takes blood tests, has shown me on a screen connected to a microscope such an undigested piece in the blood of a vegan patient. I was shocked to see that whenever this tiny undigested piece touched red blood cells, those cells instantly died. Eventually this piece of undigested food ended up being encircled in several layers of about a hundred dead cells. People who lack stomach acid end up having lots of such toxic matter circulating in their bodies. This is how a deficit of stomach acid can turn nourishing foods into harmful substances. Moreover, improper chewing combined with the lack of necessary concentration of hydrochloric acid leads to multiple nutritional deficiencies. According to Dr. James Howenstine, MD,[5] one of the main causes of insufficient stomach acid is a deficiency in zinc. As the lack of stomach acid further escalates the deficiency of zinc and other vital minerals, a vicious cycle begins.

Blending is similar to chewing, and therefore eating highly nutritious food in blended form can make a dramatic improvement to our health. After being broken down in a blender, pieces of food become the optimal size for assimilation. Liquefied greens deliver zinc and other essential nutrients to the body in an easily absorbable form regardless of hydrochloric acid levels. Consequently, deficiencies reverse and stomach acid normalizes.

For many years I couldn't understand why some people quickly lose too much weight on a raw food diet. These people have a hard time staying on a raw food diet because they feel uncomfortable living their lives with constant remarks from their friends and relatives about being too thin. I agree that humans shouldn't be too skinny. After doing a lot of research about the impact of hypochlorhydria on the assimilation of food, I asked some of my friends with this weight problem if they had ever checked their stomach acid level. Several of them got back to me and reported that they were diagnosed with very low or no stomach acid at all. Their doctors prescribed HCl pills to take with their meals. A close friend has been trying to eat raw for several years and became so thin that her husband became concerned for her health. She went to a doctor and was diagnosed with achlorhydria (no stomach acid). Her doctor put her on HCl pills, and she continued her raw food diet. She gained back several pounds and now maintains a healthy weight.

In order for nutrients to be absorbed, the food has to be broken down in the stomach both mechanically and with acids into very small pieces of 1–2 mm (0.04–0.08 inches). Raw fruits and vegetables have the most valuable nutrients in them, but they are especially hard to digest because their tough cellulose structure has to be ruptured in order to get all the nutrients out. If there is not enough stomach acid, the body is unable to receive all the nutrients it needs, including proteins, and deficiencies start to develop. I have encountered several people with such a problem who felt as if they were trapped. While eating only raw food they were able to eliminate symptoms of certain illnesses that they had, but they became very skinny. These people would then add cooked food to their diet to gain their desired weight, but their unwanted symptoms would return. Puzzled, they kept going back and forth, not knowing what to do.

That is why I felt great joy when, after teaching a couple of classes about green smoothies, I began receiving letters like this one:

> Though the raw food took care of my arthritis, I was never able to stick to it longer than two months, because on raw foods alone I dropped weight so quickly, down to 135 pounds, that my wife panicked, thinking that I was getting ill, so I had to go back to cooked foods, which made my arthritis return. When I started drinking green smoothies, my weight stabilized! I have been raw now for six months and keep my normal weight of 155 pounds. Thank you! —N. H., Canada

I have already witnessed many cases in which people with digestive problems were able to greatly improve their assimilation by adding blended greens to their diets. While cooking makes food softer and easier to digest, in the process of heating, most essential vitamins and enzymes are destroyed. Blending is a lot less harmful than cooking because it saves all the vital nutrients in the food.

Numerous conditions are associated with low stomach acidity.[6] These are just some of them: bacterial overgrowth, chronic candidiasis, parasites, Addison's disease, multiple sclerosis, arthritis, asthma, autoimmune disorders, celiac disease, stomach carcinoma, depression, dermatitis, diabetes, eczema, flatulence, gall bladder disease, gastric polyps, gastritis, hepatitis, hyperthyroidism, myasthenia gravis, osteoporosis, psoriasis, rosacea, ulcerative colitis, urticaria, and vitiligo. This is why the famous researcher Dr. Theodore A. Baroody states in his wonderful book *Alkalize or Die,* "Hydrochloric acid is absolutely essential for life."[7] In other words, no one can be completely healthy without normal levels of hydrochloric acid.

Don't confuse acidity in the stomach with alkalinity of the blood. Our blood must be slightly alkaline, and we will discuss this in upcoming chapters. "Hydrochloric acid is the *only* acid that our body produces. All other acids are by-products of metabolism and are eliminated as soon as possible."[8]

11

The Roseburg Study

When I became aware of the important functions of hydrochloric acid, I decided to perform a study. Based on the symptoms of low stomach acid that I gathered from different medical articles, I created the following questionnaire. I then printed a thousand copies and distributed them among my students. The results were shocking: I have calculated that 98.5 percent of people who answered my questionnaire had some symptoms of low stomach acidity. I invite you to check if you might have any indications of hypochlorhydria yourself.

Signs and Symptoms of Low Stomach Acidity
Read the question and check the appropriate box on the right.

	NEVER	SOMETIMES	FREQUENTLY
Do you have bloating, belching, or flatulence immediately after meals?	☐	☐	☐
Do you have indigestion, diarrhea, or constipation?	☐	☐	☐
Do you feel soreness, burning, or dryness of the mouth?	☐	☐	☐

	NEVER	SOMETIMES	FREQUENTLY
Do you have heartburn?	☐	☐	☐
Do you have multiple food allergies?	☐	☐	☐
Do you feel nauseous after taking supplements?	☐	☐	☐
Do you experience rectal itching?	☐	☐	☐
Do you have weak, peeling, and/or cracked fingernails?	☐	☐	☐
Do you have redness or dilated blood vessels in the cheeks and nose?	☐	☐	☐
Do you have adult acne?	☐	☐	☐
This question is only for women: do you experience hair loss?	☐	☐	☐
Do you have an iron deficiency?	☐	☐	☐
Do you have undigested food in the stools?	☐	☐	☐
Do you have chronic yeast infections?	☐	☐	☐
Do you have a low tolerances for dentures?	☐	☐	☐

These symptoms can be indicators of hypochlorhydria. If you have marked several symptoms even in the "sometimes" column, you may want to check your stomach acidity at the doctor's office.

I spoke to a medical doctor from Russia and was intrigued to discover how they test for hypochlorhydria there. They ask people to drink a quarter cup of beet juice and watch to see if the color of their stool or urine changes even slightly to the color of a beet. If it changes, then yes, your stomach acid is low. I was so amazed at this because I believed that such a change of color was normal for everyone, as it always was for me. However, a few months after starting to drink green smoothies, my family ate a big delicious beet salad and none of us saw that change in color anymore! Since I could only attribute such a dramatic change to drinking green smoothies, I assumed that our hydrochloric acid level had improved. In order to obtain more solid proof of this, I began planning a study that would show the effect of green smoothies on stomach acid. I wanted to find several people who were diagnosed with low hydrochloric acid and would volunteer to add green smoothies to their diets for a period of time. After they finished this smoothie trial, they would be tested again.

By some magical coincidence, as I was praying to find a doctor who would be willing to help me with such a study, one sunny morning a physician named Dr. Paul Fieber called me from Roseburg, Oregon. He told me that he and his wife had recently adopted the raw food lifestyle and needed guidance. He also shared that he had recently become disturbed by the fact that a great number of people had low stomach acid. We met the next morning to discuss our experiment in detail. Dr. Fieber became very interested in participating. The following week, Igor and I drove 120 miles to Roseburg to teach a nutrition class. After my lecture, twenty-seven people stepped forward and offered to volunteer to drink one quart of freshly made green smoothie, in addition to their regular mainstream American diet, each day for one month.

This project started on April 29, 2005. My whole family took turns blending many gallons of the green drink. To increase variety, we used any fruits and greens we could get hold of. For the entire month, all three of our local organic grocery stores were sold out of greens, mangoes, and bananas. Igor drove the valuable load 240 miles round-trip every other day. It was quite a commitment, not only for my family but also for all the people participating and even for their families. None of my dear participants ever missed a day to come to the pickup site. When I thanked this new family of mine (I call them "my in-raws") for being so dedicated and disciplined, they replied that they all felt the urgent importance of this experiment and were excited to help. Besides, many of them wanted to improve their stomach condition by natural means.

The following section describes Dr. Fieber's side of the story.

DR. PAUL'S STORY

Meeting Victoria and her family was a wonderful experience. It was amazing how fate brought us together. My wife and I were looking for help on our path to improve our health through raw food, and Victoria needed help with her study.

There are different methods of testing HCl, but we decided that the HCl challenge test would work out best for us, considering our timeline. The HCl challenge test is designed to help determine the ability of the stomach to produce adequate stomach acid. The body has evolved to release stomach acid in response to appropriate stimuli. Thinking about food, chewing, and the presence of certain foods (healthy or not) in the stomach, for example proteins, milk, calcium salts, and coffee, stimulate the release of gastrin, a hormone secreted by gastrin cells, or G cells, in the pyloric glands located in the antrum of the stomach. Gastrin strongly stimulates the parietal glands to produce and secrete acid into the stomach. Histamine is another hormone that stimulates acid production. Its effect is potentiated by the presence of gastrin. Many people have a deficient acid-producing process and suffer from hypochlorhydria, or in more serious cases, achlorhydria.

Many of my patients complain of gastric reflux due to "excess" stomach acid secretion. In my experience, hypersecretion of stomach acid is not common. Inappropriate timing of stomach acid, however, is common and can produce symptoms in an irritated or inflamed digestive tract. For many, reflux of stomach contents into the esophagus has more to do with inadequate secretions of stomach acid leading to the putrefaction of food and the accompanying symptoms of gas, bloating, reflux, and belching. Antacid therapy may provide temporary relief but does nothing to get to the cure.

In our study, each participant was given ten HCl capsules, which were enough to "challenge" four meals. We asked our group to challenge meals that were high in protein and were substantial, complex meals. They started with one capsule with the first meal, and if they had no mild burning or irritation, they were to increase to two capsules with the next meal and continue until they had a reaction or reached a total of four capsules with no reaction at all. Out of the twenty-seven participants, only two people had a reaction with one capsule, and at that time they discontinued the study. The rest of our group all had some degree of hypochlorhydria and went on to participate in the study. Their ages ranged from seventeen to eighty. All the participants were asked not to change any other part of their diet.

After thirty days of drinking one quart of green smoothie each day, we then completed another HCl challenge test to see what improvement occurred over the month. One person dropped out in the middle of the study due to nausea. Out of the other twenty-four participants, we had sixteen of the group who showed improvement in their production of HCl. It was remarkable to me that 66.7 percent of the participants showed such vast improvement. I did not expect to see this much progress in such a short period of time. The fiber content and nutrient value of the green smoothies made for an incredible success. All the participants also noted many other improvements in their health, some of which were dramatic changes.

I would also like to give my own personal testimonial, as my wife and I had been drinking green smoothies for about two months before the study was conducted. My blood pressure, pulse rate, and cholesterol readings all improved substantially. We lost all cravings for cooked food, and the green smoothies were both delicious and fulfilling. The most significant change for me concerned a small growth that had appeared on my nose. After one month on the green smoothies, the growth fell off and left a small hole where it had been. This proved to me the tremendous healing properties of the green smoothie.

I would like to personally thank Victoria for providing me the opportunity to contribute to such a remarkable study. I have met very few people in my life who have been as dedicated and have had such a passion for helping others. Thank you, Victoria; you have changed our lives forever.

■ ■ ■

As Dr. Fieber mentions, we were expecting some positive changes, but we didn't know they would be so significant in such a short period of time. Most experiments like this one usually run for three to six months but since the cost was out of our own pockets, we did only what we could afford. The Roseburg Experiment demonstrated that regular consumption of green smoothies greatly benefits people's health through improving their hydrochloric acid levels. Therefore, consumers of green smoothies should expect:

- to have better absorption of valuable nutrients;
- to lessen the possibility of infection and parasites;
- to heal allergies;
- to improve overall health.

Better absorption is in itself a great advantage. For example, better absorption of calcium may decrease the chance of osteoporosis, better absorption of iron may help to heal anemia, better absorption of B vitamins may protect against nerve disorders, and so on.

After consuming green smoothies for just one month, Roseburg Study participants noted the following health improvements in addition to improved stomach acid: increased energy, depression lifted and suicidal thoughts gone, less blood sugar fluctuation, more regular bowel movements, dandruff cleared up, no more insomnia, asthma attacks stopped completely, none of the usual PMS symptoms, stronger fingernails, fewer coffee cravings, sex life improved, skin cleared up, and many more. It was interesting to see that most of the participants who wanted to lose weight lost anywhere from five to ten pounds, and a couple of people who wanted to gain weight were able to gain one or two pounds.

The participants of the Roseburg Study were so excited about their results that some rumors got back to me that they were considering changing the name of their town to Raws'burg!

The fact that all of the healing qualities of green smoothies were proven by practical experimentation makes this simple drink truly special. I am hoping to inspire as many people as possible to incorporate green smoothies into their everyday lives.

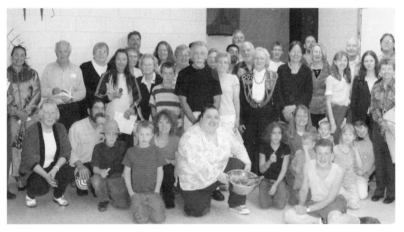

Raws'burg group with their families and friends

12

Greens Make the Body More Alkaline

I feel that in our search for health we have been treading in the same place for many decades. In the meantime the most prevalent illness, cancer, is getting worse every year. Let's look at the statistics for 2005.[1]

- It is estimated that 1,372,910 new cancer cases and 570,260 cancer deaths occurred; five-year survival rates rose from 50 to 74 percent from the 1970s
- Lung cancer remained the biggest killer, estimated to claim the lives of 163,510 people.
- About 232,090 men were diagnosed with prostate cancer, which killed 30,350.
- Some 211,240 women were diagnosed with breast cancer, which killed 40,410.

I have observed, first in Russia and later in the United States, that mainstream medicine seems to have been focusing on the secondary causes of disease. To me that's like pushing a car that has run out of gas with your bare hands instead of putting gas in it, or comforting a hungry person instead of feeding them. So what is the main cause of disease?

Today we have an ocean of confusing information, including articles in which different experts state many different reasons for illness. However, I think the main reason for illness was stated very clearly in 1931. Over eighty years ago, Otto Warburg was awarded the Nobel Prize for his discovery that cancer is caused by weakened cell respiration due to a lack of oxygen at the cellular level. According to Warburg, damaged cell respiration causes fermentation, resulting in low pH (acidity) at the cellular level.

Dr. Warburg, in his Nobel Prize–winning study, illustrated the environment of the cancer cell. A normal healthy cell undergoes an adverse change when it can no longer take in oxygen to convert glucose into energy. In the absence of oxygen, the cell reverts to a primal nutritional program to nourish itself by converting glucose through the process of fermentation. The lactic acid produced by fermentation lowers the cell's pH (acid-alkaline balance) and destroys the ability of DNA and RNA to control cell division. The cancer cells then begin to multiply. The lactic acid simultaneously causes severe local pain as it destroys cell enzymes. Cancer appears as a rapidly growing external cell covering with a core of dead cells.

Dr. Otto Warburg finished one of his most famous speeches with the following statement: "Nobody today can say that one does not know what cancer and its prime cause is. On the contrary, there is no disease whose prime cause is better known, so that today ignorance is no longer an excuse that one cannot do more about prevention."[2]

Otto Warburg won the Nobel Prize for showing that cancer thrives in anaerobic (without oxygen), or acidic, conditions. In other words, the main cause of cancer is acidity of the human body. By the time I read his genius speech, he had been dead a long time.

I wondered, if this discovery was so important that he received the Nobel Prize, why doesn't everyone know what pH is?

As soon as scientists discovered what healthy human blood pressure and temperature were supposed to be, devices were invented to measure them. Whenever I went to a doctor, my blood pressure and temperature were measured, but I don't ever remember a doctor measuring my pH. High blood pressure and fever, though not pleasant, do not cause cancer. The acidic condition of the blood does. This is what the internationally renowned scientist Dr. Warburg has proven. Therefore it seems vital to make pH information immediately available to everyone.

It makes great sense to me that children should study the pH index of all foods at school and that all foods sold to the public should have their pH index printed on the content label together with calories and nutrients. For example, Parmesan cheese should have a red warning label with a pH sign saying it is extremely acid forming, at -34, while spinach would have a golden medal sign with a pH index of +14, as an excellent alkalizing food. The pH indexes have been measured in biochemical laboratories and cannot be guessed just by looking at foods. Some foods are surprisingly alkaline or acidic; for example, most people are amazed to learn that the lemon is one of the most alkalizing fruits, while walnuts are slightly acidifying. I think it's important for the U.S. Department of Agriculture's food pyramid to reflect the pH of different foods as soon as possible. I imagine that many people's health could instantly be improved by their ability to consume alkalizing foods that are more beneficial for human health. You can find a complete list of pH values of different foods in the book *The pH Miracle* by Robert Young.

It is a popular delusion among dieters that fats are the single contributor to weight gain. This misconception leads to massive confusion and explains why so many overweight people are not succeeding in losing weight. I am sure that many people would be shocked to find out that we may gain weight from eating, say, cheese not only because it is rich in fat but mostly due to its high pH acid level. In response to high pH acid, the body creates fat cells to store the acid. For example, almonds have 70 percent fat, and pork has only 58 percent. However, pork has one of the highest acid values, -38, while almonds are alkaline forming, at +3.[3] This is why it is so crucial to know, in addition to nutritional values, the pH index—to have it available and handy at every store, printed on each food label, showing its ability to alkalize the body. Knowing the pH indexes of various foods can help us balance our personal daily meal plans.

I remember how my mother was in tears in 1965 after reading an article in a Russian health magazine that stated that watermelons and cucumbers do not have any nutritional value. They were our family's favorite foods. Forty years later, I am learning that cucumbers and watermelons are so alkalizing that they can neutralize the acidifying effect of eating beef. I am glad that my parents continued to buy watermelons, despite "scientific" recommendations.

Many years ago, back in Russia, when I was studying to be a medical nurse, our professor told us that the cholesterol in our food did not contribute to the cholesterol level in our blood because it was our own liver that made cholesterol. Therefore, I was not surprised or disappointed by the diet high in fat and animal protein that my father was receiving while staying at the cardio center. After my dad's massive heart attack, they served him beefsteak with gravy and milk. Later, after reading a lot of books and articles about the importance of the proper pH balance in the body, I understood that the so-called "bad" cholesterol, lipoprotein (LDL), is made by our own liver in order to bind the toxins and deactivate the acidic waste that comes from certain foods, such as fats and animal protein. Unfortunately, I bought my first book on this topic, *Alkalize or Die,*[4] two months after my father died from his second heart attack.

Food is not the only factor that affects our pH balance. Any stress can potentially leave an acidic residue in our body; conversely, any activities that are calming and relaxing can make us more alkaline.

Factors that potentially make us more acidic include hearing or saying harsh or bitter words, loud music and noise, being in a traffic jam, feeling jealousy or wanting revenge, grieving, hearing a baby crying, overworking and overexercising, beginning or finishing school, going on vacation, watching scary or stressful movies, watching and listening to TV, talking on the phone for a long time, taking on a mortgage, paying bills and credit cards, and so on.

Factors that potentially make us more alkaline include giving or receiving a smile or a hug, laughter and jokes, classical or quiet music, seeing a puppy, hearing a compliment or blessing, receiving a soft massage, staying in a cozy and clean environment, being in nature, watching children laugh and play, walking and sleeping under the stars and moonlight, working in the garden, observing flowers, singing or playing a musical instrument, sincere friendly conversation, and many others.

I find it helpful to observe my body's inner reaction to different events around me and if I notice unwanted feeling of stress, I try to make changes not only to my diet but to my whole way of living.

Being uneducated about pH balance breeds a lot of confusion among people who are looking for healthy diets. They try many different things, very often without positive results. For example, in my own experience, I have been eating only raw food for many years. While this was a vast improvement over my previous diet, I did not reach the optimal results I desired because I did not consume enough greens. I read several books and articles on the subject of pH balance and bought litmus paper with which to measure my pH. However, every time I measured my saliva or urine, it was almost always acid. So I got even more confused and stopped measuring. I was convinced that my diet was the best it could be because what could be better than a raw food diet? I didn't understand the importance of keeping the proper alkaline balance in my body.

Once I started drinking green smoothies, I decided to check my pH balance again. I tested both my saliva and urine and was surprised to see that my litmus paper was now the stable green color of alkalinity!

As soon as I clearly noticed the tight connection between our food intake and pH balance, I purchased plenty of pH tape (litmus paper) for my family and placed it in the bathrooms and kitchens, available at any time, so we could check our pH balance every day and rest assured that our health was out of danger. After being on a one-hundred-percent raw diet for so many years, I have come to the conclusion that *it is impossible to maintain a good alkaline pH balance without consuming large quantities of dark leafy greens,* approximately one to two bunches, or one to one-and-a-half pounds every day. Some people try to keep a normal pH balance by taking supplements containing dried greens. While this is certainly better than eating only French fries, I strongly believe that consuming fresh greens is thousands of times better because supplements are processed food and their nutritional content is altered, causing loss of nutrients. Also, when consumed in the form of capsules and tablets, they enter our body in huge concentrated doses, and any additional nutrients create extra work for the elimination system. Once when I was visiting a friend who was a horse trainer, my daughter and I conducted an interesting experiment. We wanted to find out if the horses preferred dry hay or fresh greens. We both took excellent quality hay in one hand and freshly gathered weeds in the other. Six out of six horses preferred the fresh greens over the quality hay. In nature, animals instinctively always go for the freshest option.

Out of all the choices that we have in consuming greens, the green smoothie is a winner because it is a complete food, it is fresh, and it takes less than a minute to prepare.

13

Healthy Soil Is More Valuable than Gold

We are the dust of the earth.
—DR. BERNARD JENSEN

When I read my first book on permaculture, a natural way of gardening, I unexpectedly learned such stunning facts about soil that I have radically changed many of my habits. In addition to composting, recycling, and buying only organic food, I now have a small permaculture garden of my own. Most importantly, I have developed a deep respect for all soils.

During the hundreds of millions of years that plants have been living on our planet, they have become amazingly self-sufficient. In addition to establishing a useful relationship with the sun, plants have learned to "grow" their own soil. When plants die, it may look to us like they just fall on the ground and rot, getting eaten by multitudes of bugs and worms. However, researchers were shocked to discover that dead plants get consumed only by particular bacteria and fungi.[1] Plants "know" how to attract to their own rotting only those microorganisms and earthworms that will produce beneficial minerals for the soil where the plants' siblings will grow. One way plants attract particular microorganisms into their soil is by concentrating more sugars in their roots. Thus roots such as carrots and potatoes are always much sweeter than the rest of the plant. Plants and microorganisms develop a symbiotic relationship that is beneficial to both plant and microbe.[2] Just like humans with our farm animals, plants "breed" certain microorganisms and specific kinds of fungi that produce the humus (organic matter) that is rich in the most useful minerals for these plants. Apparently, the quality of the soil is critically important, not only as a source of water and minerals for plants but for their very survival. That is why plants must never be researched separately from the soil they grow in.

If we care which nutrients we receive from plants, we absolutely cannot ignore the quality of nutrients plants receive from the soil because *we literally consume minerals from the soil through plants.* The quality of the soil in which plants grow has an immense influence on the health of the people and animals that eat those plants. The following example with purebred horses clearly demonstrates the impact soil can have on people and animals:

> Within a few generations, the originally giant dappled Percheron draft horses, developed on the soils of a French district south of Normandy, had dwindled to the size of Cossack horses, though their bloodlines had been kept pure by the Soviets and their confirmation remained the same, though miniaturized.[3]

This case reveals that the soils plants grow in are as important to our health as the plants themselves, if not more so. In other words, as odd as it sounds, *our well-being depends on the quality of the land in which our food grows because the original source of nutrients for humans comes from soils, not plants.*

The main difference between organic and conventional gardening is that "Conventional agriculture attempts to feed the plants while the organic method nourishes the microorganisms in soil."[4] In other words, conventional farmers ignore the microorganisms in the soil and aim their efforts at supplying potassium, nitrogen, and other chemicals for the sake of plants, while organic gardeners take care of feeding the living things in the soil that provide harmoniously balanced nutrients to the plants. Just as humans cannot live on chemicals instead of food, microorganisms in the soil cannot survive when fed artificial fertilizers. When all microorganisms get destroyed with chemicals, the soil turns to dust. No plants can grow in dust, no matter how rich in various chemicals this dust is.

Through the plants we eat, we receive essential nutrients that were broken down by microorganisms in the soil. The more organic matter, or humus, is in the soil, the more nutritious is the food grown in this soil.

There is growing scientific evidence of the superiority of organic food in comparison to conventionally grown food. In a major, in-depth review[1] of the scientific literature on this subject, a group of researchers identified 236 scientifically valid measurements of organic and conventional samples of produce. After thorough evaluation of gathered data, scientists concluded: "The average serving of organic plant-based food contains about 25% more of the nutrients encompassed in this study than a comparable-sized serving of the same food produced by conventional farming methods."

Plants seem to be much better "farmers" than we are. As a result of their clever "gardening" for millions of years, we humans have inherited many feet of beautiful, fruitful topsoil all around the globe with zillions of happy microorganisms thriving in it. In their best-selling book, *Secrets of the Soil,* Peter Tompkins and Christopher Bird state that "the combined weight of all the microbial cells on earth is twenty-five times that of its animal life; every acre of well-cultivated land contains up to a half a ton of thriving microorganisms, and a ton of earthworms which can daily excrete a ton of humic castings."[6]

As a result of our "highly technological" human gardening, most of the soil of agricultural farms in the United States contains less than 2 percent of organic matter, while originally, before the era of chemistry, it was 60 to 90 percent. According to David Blume, an ecological biologist and permaculture teacher and expert, "Most Class I commercial agricultural soil is lucky to hit 2 percent organic matter—the dividing line between a living and dead soil."[7] By applying permaculture gardening techniques to a field of extremely depleted soil, which consisted of cement-hard adobe clay, David Blume was able to bring the organic matter up to the 25 percent level within a couple of years. From this field he harvested the crops "eight times what the USDA claims are possible per square foot."[8]

We cannot successfully feed soils with chemicals because "biology does not equal chemistry."[9] In other words, chemical fertilizers are missing live enzymes that contribute to the most unique qualities of all soils. According to the abundance of research done in different countries, soil enzymes can transform one element into another if such "biological transmutation" would benefit the plants that grow in this soil. Take a look at the following quotes from numerous studies and see for yourself.

Professor René Furon of the Faculty of Sciences at Paris University states, "It can no longer be denied that nature makes magnesium out of calcium (in some cases the reverse takes place); that potassium can come from sodium."[10]

Hisatoki Komaki, head of a biological research laboratory at the Matsushita Electric Company in Japan, states, "Various microorganisms, including certain bacteria and two species each of molds and yeasts, were capable of transmuting sodium into potassium."[11]

Professor P. A. Korolkov in Russia states, "silicon can be converted to aluminum. ... We are being subjected to a radical revision, not of minutiae, but of the basic status of an inherited natural science. The time has come to recognize that any chemical element can turn into another, under natural conditions."[12]

These are the solid facts from which we can conclude that chemical fertilizers could never enrich the living soil but can only damage or even destroy it with the most devastating consequences for plants, animals, and people.

14

The Healing Powers of Chlorophyll

The moment one gives close attention to anything, even a blade of grass, it becomes a mysterious, awesome, indescribably magnificent world in itself.
—HENRY MILLER

The longer I live, the more I admire nature. When hiking in the morning, if I run into a deer, squirrel, or any other creature, I freeze and absorb them with my eyes zealously, as if nothing else matters for me. I sense a great mystery in animals, flowers, trees, and especially in the sun. When I look at the sun, I appreciate that sunshine is free and equally available to everyone.

Many people enjoy the sun. We all feel better and look healthier if we regularly spend time in the sun. We attempt to get as much sunlight as possible. Our bathing suits have become reduced to the very minimum as we try to immerse our bodies in the precious sunshine. However, not many people are aware of sunlight's liquefied form, chlorophyll.

Chlorophyll is as important as sunlight! No life is possible without sunshine, and no life is possible without chlorophyll. Chlorophyll is liquefied sun energy. Consuming as much chlorophyll as possible is like bathing our inner organs in sunshine. The molecule of chlorophyll is remarkably similar to the heme molecule in human blood.[1] Chlorophyll takes care of our body like a most caring and loving mother. It heals and cleanses all our organs and even destroys many of our internal enemies, like pathogenic bacteria, fungi, cancer cells,[2] and many others.

To experience optimal health we need to have 80 to 85 percent of "good" bacteria in our intestines. Friendly bacteria manufacture many essential nutrients for our body, including vitamin K, B vitamins, numerous helpful enzymes, and other vital substances. Such "good," or aerobic, bacteria thrive in the presence of oxygen and require it for their continued growth and existence. That is why, if we do not have enough oxygen in the cells of our body, "bad" bacteria take over and begin to thrive, causing an extreme amount of infection and disease. These pathogenic bacteria are anaerobic and cannot tolerate gaseous oxygen. Taking care of our intestinal flora is vitally important. "Good" bacteria can easily be destroyed by countless factors, including antibiotics, poor diet, overeating, and stress. In this case, we could have 80 to 90 percent of "bad" bacteria filling our body with toxic acidic waste. I believe that the dominance of anaerobic bacteria in our intestines is one of the prime causes of all disease.

Since ancient times, chlorophyll has served as a miraculous healer. Chlorophyll carries significant amounts of oxygen with it and thus plays a critical role in supporting the aerobic bacteria. Therefore, the more chlorophyll we consume, the better our intestinal flora and overall health will be. Considering that greens are a major source of chlorophyll, it is difficult to find a better way of consuming chlorophyll than drinking green smoothies.

Chlorophyll has been proven helpful in preventing and healing many forms of cancer[3] and arteriosclerosis.[4] Abundant scientific research shows that there are hardly any illnesses that could not be helped by chlorophyll. In order to describe all the remedial qualities of chlorophyll, I would have to write a whole separate volume. So I have listed only some of the many healing properties of this amazing substance.

Chlorophyll:

- builds a high red blood cell count
- helps prevent cancer
- provides iron to organs
- makes the body more alkaline
- counteracts toxins eaten
- improves anemic conditions
- cleans and deodorizes bowel tissues
- helps purify the liver
- aids hepatitis improvement
- regulates menstruation
- aids hemophilia condition
- improves milk production
- helps sores heal faster
- eliminates body odors
- resists bacteria in wounds
- cleans tooth and gum structure in pyorrhea
- eliminates bad breath
- relieves sore throat
- makes an excellent oral surgery gargle
- benefits inflamed tonsils
- soothes ulcer tissues
- soothes painful hemorrhoids and piles
- aids catarrhal discharges
- revitalizes vascular system in the legs
- improves varicose veins
- reduces pain caused by inflammation
- improves vision

The most important goal of all life-forms on our planet is the continuation of their life. What do we humans need to survive? Besides air and water, our primary need is food. We get our food from plants and animals. Where do plants get their food? Plants obtain their food from the soil and directly from the sun. Only plants "know" how to convert sunlight into carbohydrates. Plants use these carbohydrates for various functions. A portion of the sugar goes to the fruit in order to attract animals, birds, humans, and other beings to help spread their seeds. A large part of the sugar made from chlorophyll is transferred to the plant's roots. As you know, the roots of plants have a sweet taste: for example, carrots, beets, yams, potatoes, and turnips. There are countless varieties of fungi, microbes, amoebas, bacteria, and other microorganisms whose lives depend on the sugar in plant roots. Also, plants use carbohydrates to build new stems, roots, and bark, and, most importantly, they build new leaves because leaves can make more carbohydrates. This is why the mass of leaves is always greater in relation to the rest of the plant. Since green plants are always trying to increase absorption of chlorophyll, they continuously keep growing, and as a result we constantly have to trim the bushes and cut the grass around our homes; otherwise they would keep growing without stopping until they took over the entire space, leaving no room for us.

Plants' lives depend on sunshine, and our life depends on plants. Even when people eat animals they eat them for the sake of the nutrients that the animal received earlier through consuming plants. That is why humans almost never eat carnivorous animals but only the ones that eat plants. Ancient teachings of Judaism, Islam, and other religions prohibit the eating of carnivorous animals like lions, tigers, leopards, foxes, eagles, and pelicans. My grandmother recalled that during the war, when her hungry relatives tried eating the meat of carnivorous animals and birds, they all became violently ill. At the same time, no living creatures, even carnivores, could survive without consuming some greens. We all notice how dogs and cats occasionally eat green grass.

With the high oxygen content in chlorophyll and the high mineral content in green plants, greens are the most alkalizing food that exists on our planet. By including green smoothies in our diet, we can keep our bodies alkaline and healthy.

Another great way to get chlorophyll and nutrients from greens is drinking wheatgrass juice. This highly nourishing drink was invented by Dr. Ann Wigmore and is becoming more and more popular all the time. Wheatgrass juice consists of 70 percent chlorophyll and contains 92 different minerals of the 102 minerals in the human body, as well as beta carotene, the B vitamins, vitamins C, E, H, and K, 19 amino acids, and beneficial enzymes. All of these properties make wheatgrass an extraordinary health builder.

However, the strong nutritional density of wheatgrass juice makes it hard for many people to drink. Many would like to consume it regularly but cannot do so because of nauseous reactions sometimes caused by the smell alone. I also tried many times to start drinking wheatgrass and could not keep it down even after learning the special "wheatgrass dance," saying a special prayer, clipping my nose, and other tricks.

After drinking green smoothies regularly for one year, I was offered a shot of wheatgrass and, unexpectedly, I loved it. Now for the first time in my life I am able to comfortably drink four, six, eight, or more ounces of wheatgrass each day. I was so amazed and pleased that for a while I continued to visit our local Ashland Co-op to drink wheatgrass, paying $10 to $15 at a time just for this drink. I heard the girls that work at the juice bar telling each other that they had never seen anybody drinking so much of it so easily. None of them could drink any wheatgrass at all. These days I don't consume it daily but if I have a chance, I always go for it. I think that this dramatic change in my body's acceptance of wheatgrass has to do with my improved level of stomach acid.

The Wisdom of Plants

We have already discussed the sophisticated relationship plants have with soil and sunshine. Apparently, millions of years of coexistence on the same planet has resulted in plants, people, and animals developing strong symbiotic connections. Plants do not mind if people and animals eat their fruits because this practice benefits the plant by spreading its seeds for future generations. In fact, plants are "interested" in someone eating their fruit, but only when it is ripe. As I stated before, the goal of all plants is the continuation of their species and providing adequate living conditions for them. That is why nearly all the fruits in the world have a round shape, so that they can roll away and start a new life. For the very same reason, plants have learned to make their fruit colorful, palatable, and nutritious to ensure that their consumers not only eat one fruit but continue to return for more. This strategy works very well, and all fruit gets eaten. Have you ever noticed how thoroughly birds "clean" cherry trees or how squirrels keep working on an oak tree until there are no more acorns left? What happens next? The eaters digest their food, have bowel movements far away from the mother plant, and the seeds are covered with nice organic fertilizer. The seeds get a perfect start. Inside the fruit, the seeds are wisely protected from being digested with hardy shells and inhibitors. Note that the plant keeps its fruit extremely untasteful, colorless, and without attractive fragrance all the way until the seeds are ripe so that nobody wastes them before the seeds have matured.

The following example illustrates how much the continuation of their species means to plants. In a recent study in Russia, biologists discovered that:

> When a tree is foreseeing its death, the tree gathers its entire energy and deposits this energy into producing seeds for the very last time. For example, the oak tree broken by a storm or the cedar tree with its bark removed from its trunk, in a farewell effort before they die forever, give their record crops of acorns or nuts.[1]

In contrast with this example, when a plant is genetically altered, it does not produce seeds on purpose. Such a plant makes itself infertile to prevent future unhealthy generations. Seedless watermelons are usually odorless and tasteless because an upset plant has no motivation to make its fruits sweet, fragrant, or attractive in any other way. I am sure that it is not healthy to eat seedless plants because their entire chemistry, electromagnetic charge, and who knows what else, has been altered. In my own life, I prefer to pay double for an organic seeded watermelon or grapes.

Plants don't want us to eat their trunk and roots. That is why the roots are hidden in the ground. The roots are for the microorganisms in the soil, as described in the previous chapter. The trunk is purposely covered with hard and bitter bark. With greens, plants demonstrate their perfect ability to develop symbiosis with different creatures. Plants "allow" humans and animals to eat all of their fruits, but only part of their leaves, because plants need to have leaves for their own use—which is manufacturing chlorophyll. At the same time, plants depend on moving creatures for many different reasons, such as pollination, fertilizing the soil, and hanging around to help eat the ripe fruit. However, if, for example, a deer eats all the green leaves off a lilac bush, the plant will inevitably die. To prevent this, nature placed a minute amount of alkaloids (poisons) in every green leaf on earth. That is how animals are forced to rotate their menu, and that is why all wild animals are browsers. They eat a small amount of one kind of leaf, then move on to many other plants during the course of the day. The amount of alkaloids in a single plant is minute and is healthy, as it strengthens the immune system. This principle became the basis of the science of homeopathy. However, one has to be careful not to accumulate larger amounts of alkaloids by continuously eating the same plant over a long period of time. For this reason, we humans need to rotate our greens as much as possible instead of eating only, for example, iceberg lettuce and romaine. From my experience, if I use at least seven different greens, I don't have any problems. Usually I rotate the following greens on a regular basis: kale, chard, spinach, parsley, dandelion greens, romaine, cilantro, and a variety of lettuces. In the summer I significantly increase my variety.

Chimpanzees also rotate the green plants they eat. They go through approximately 117 different plants in one year.[2] I was able to locate only about forty types of various greens, including edible weeds, that are available in my state, Oregon. I hope that our farmers will learn to grow a larger assortment of green leafy vegetables to increase our green sources. The following is a list of greens that my family has been rotating in our diet during the last year.

Greens

arugula	escarole	
asparagus	frisée	
beet greens (tops)	kale (three types)	
bok choy	mizuna	
broccoli	mustard greens	
carrot tops	radicchio	
celery	radish tops	
chard	romaine lettuce, green	
collard greens	and red leaves (no iceberg	
edible flowers	or light-colored leaves)	
endive	spinach	

Weeds

chickweed
clover
dandelion (greens
    and flowers)
lambsquarters
mallow *(Malva)*
miner's lettuce
plantain
purslane
stinging nettles

Herbs

aloe vera	parsley (two types)
baby dill	peppermint leaves
basil	spearmint
cilantro	
fennel	
mint	

Sprouts

alfalfa
broccoli
clover
fenugreek
radish
sunflower

Wild edibles often contain more vitamins and minerals than commercially marketed plants. Weeds have not been "spoiled" by farmers' care in contrast to the "good" plants of the garden. In order to survive in spite of constant weeding, pulling, and spraying, weeds had to develop strong survival properties. For example, in order to stay alive without being watered, most weeds have developed unbelievably long roots. If you have ever tried to pull out a dandelion plant with its roots, you understand what I mean. Alfalfa's roots grow up to twenty feet long, reaching for the most fertile layers of the soil. As a result, all wild plants possess more nutrients than commercially grown plants. I feel so silly now when I remember how I used to always pull out the "nasty" lambsquarters from my garden to let my "precious" iceberg lettuce grow.

While there are countless benefits associated with eating wild foods, there are also some risks. It is a good idea to first learn how to positively identify edible plants. I urge you to *take caution when harvesting wild foods.* Eating wild edibles is fun, healthful, and safe when done properly. Please take the time to educate yourself and your loved ones. If you are ever in doubt about whether a plant is edible or not, please, please don't eat it!

The best way to learn which local weeds are edible is to sign up for an herb walk with an experienced guide in your area. This way you can learn to recognize particular edible plants by actually touching, smelling, and tasting them so that you can gather your "wild produce" on your own. There are lots of articles and photos of edible weeds on the Internet, and you may also find many books that help identify edible plants in your area.

For variety, we include several kinds of sprouts in our diet, but never more than a handful and only one or two times a week. From approximately the third to the sixth day of their lives, sprouts contain higher levels of alkaloids as a means of protection from animals nipping them off and killing them.[3] That doesn't mean that sprouts are poisonous or dangerous, but only that we cannot live on sprouts alone. Most sprouts are rich in B vitamins and have a hundred times more nutrients than a fully developed plant because sprouts need more nutrition for their period of rapid growth.

Once in a while I read in the news or receive an e-mail about kale or spinach or parsley or some other green having a toxic ingredient and therefore being dangerous for human consumption. This is all true, but not to such a degree that we should exclude any particular green from our diet. Let's learn to increase the variety of greens in our diet and to rotate them constantly for better nutritional results.

There are several other ways in which plants protect themselves from being destroyed. Some plants have thorns instead of alkaloids, and one type of acacia tree in Africa is inhabited by colonies of very aggressive ants with a painful sting.

Thorny plants like cactuses and stinging nettles contain significantly less or no alkaloids, which makes them a valuable addition to our diet. Of course, we first need to figure out how to eat them. I have often successfully added stinging nettles and cactuses to my green smoothies. After being processed in a high-speed blender, the spikes are usually completely blended up.

When I think about all the little tricks plants have developed for their survival, I feel an immense respect and admiration for nature. Our symbiosis with plants has developed over the course of millions of years, but we could ruin it in just a matter of decades. I believe that we still can repair our relationship with nature. Returning to our original diet is one necessary step toward this goal.

16

Greens: The Original Source of Omega-3s

The important thing is not to stop questioning.
—ALBERT EINSTEIN

What is one of the most striking differences between a humming-bird and a hibernating bear? Their metabolism. One animal moves extremely fast and the other is extremely slow, largely due to differences in the composition of fat in their bodies. According to recent scientific research on factors affecting metabolism, "the fats of high-speed animals such as the hummingbird are loaded with the omega-3 fatty acids."[1] In contrast, bears have to accumulate a lot of omega-6 fatty acids in their fat before they can go into hibernation.* Omega-3s and omega-6s are seemingly alike substances and are even united under one name: essential polyunsaturated fatty acids. However, there are major differences between them.

---

*"It's a pretty neat system. Plants respond to the changing light by making or losing leaves, and animals use their changing food supply to prepare themselves for the future. ... As animals reduce their intake of leaves (and/or animals that eat leaves) and increase their intake of seeds (and/or animals that eat seeds), seed fats come to outnumber leaf fats in the membranes of their cells. Metabolic rate falls and animals gain weight, which they store as fat. Come spring, as seeds germinate and form leaves (a process in which the omega-6s are turned into omega-3s by an enzyme that only plants have), an animal's new, green, *faster* diet prepares it for activity and reproduction." Susan Allport, *The Queen of Fats: Why Omega-3s Were Removed from the Western Diet and What We Can Do to Replace Them* (Berkeley: University of California Press, 2006).

The omega-3 molecule is unique in its ability to rapidly change its shape. This exceptional flexibility is passed to organs that absorb it. Omega-3s thin the blood of humans and animals as well as the sap of plants. As a result of these qualities, omega-3s are utilized by the fastest-functioning organs in the body. For example, omega-3s enable our hearts to beat properly, our blood to flow freely, our eyes to see, and our brains to make decisions faster and more clearly.

The omega-6 fatty acids, on the other hand, serve the opposite function: they thicken the blood of humans and animals as well as the juices of plants. Omega-6s solidify and cause inflammation of the tissues. Some scientists link an excess of omega-6s in the human diet with such conditions as heart disease, stroke, arthritis, asthma, menstrual cramps, diabetes, headaches, and tumor metastases.[2]

After I first heard about the significance of omega-3s in the human diet, I began searching for more information and read everything I could possibly find on the subject. *The Queen of Fats,* a book written by Susan Allport in 2006, has been particularly useful to me; it contains a wealth of reference material, most of which I was able to find online and research further.

According to Allport,[3] there are numerous studies looking into the role that omega-6 fats play in the promotion of certain cancers, including breast, prostate, and colon cancer, and exploring the benefits of omega-3s in treating psychological disorders such as depression and postpartum depression, attention deficit disorder, and bipolar disorder. A growing number of diseases are being associated with an imbalance of the essential fats; not just heart disease, cancer, depression, immune disorders, and arthritis but obesity and diabetes as well.

For many decades, nutritionists have been linking obesity to the overconsumption of foods high in fat, particularly in saturated fat. Since then, many people have been trying to reduce the percentage of fat in their diet. From 1955 to 1995, Americans reduced fat consumption from 40 percent of their total calorie intake to 35 percent. According to the United States Department of Agriculture (USDA), while Americans decreased their consumption of saturated fats, they increased their consumption of salad and cooking oils from 9.8 pounds per person in 1955 to 35.2 pounds per person in 2000.[4] So despite these efforts to eat healthier, the percentage of overweight adults in the U.S. during this same time period grew from 25 percent to 47 percent.[5] Apparently we have been eating the wrong fats.

When I was a little girl in Russia in the early sixties, my mother would give me a glass bottle and send me to the store to buy vegetable oil. She told me to always ask what date the oil had been delivered before I purchased any. If the oil was more than a week old, I had to go to another store. That was how quickly the freshly pressed oil could become rancid. At home, we knew to never leave the oil in direct sunlight and to store it in a dark, cool place to help keep it fresh.

By the time I had my own family, technological advances had increased the shelf life of sunflower, corn, and other vegetable oils to one year. As I understand now, such convenience had been achieved by removing omega-3s from the oil due to their highly perishable nature. As a result, over the course of several decades many of our foods have become increasingly richer in omega-6 fatty acids and deficient in omega-3s. In recent years, genetic engineers have been manipulating seeds, trying to develop strains with higher omega-6 and lower omega-3 content in order to even further prolong the storage life of seeds and the oils made from them. In addition, most farm animals, such as cattle, sheep, pigs, and chickens have increasingly been fed soy, corn, and other grains instead of grass and hay. People who consume animal products would benefit from knowing that the meat from animals that consume grass is rich in omega-3s while the meat from animals that consume corn and other grains is rich in omega-6s. Even fish are now fed grains at fish farms.[6] In nature, small fish as well as some species of whales eat phytoplankton, microscopic algae rich in chlorophyll, which is the original source for omega-3 fatty acids in fish. Larger fish eat the smaller fish and humans then catch and eat many of these larger fish,[7] which is why wild fish are famous for their high omega-3 content. Contrary to this, farmed fish often have more omega-6s than omega-3s.[8]

The same pattern appears in dairy products and eggs. For example, one study showed that eggs from free-range chickens that had feasted on grass, insects, and a very small amount of grain contained twenty times more omega-3 fatty acids than did standard supermarket eggs.[9] We've seen that one of the disadvantages of a diet rich in omega-6 fatty acids is that it slows down metabolic functions and promotes significant weight gain, as in the case of the hibernating bear. Whereas in a bear the function is a healthy cyclical one, the same is not true for humans! And the paradox of many obese people today is that they are starved for fat—they have more omega-6 than they need but are deficient in beneficial omega-3 fatty acids. Not only all chips, crackers, and cookies are made with seeds and oils but almost all salads and vegetarian dishes in restaurants are prepared with vegetable oils, loaded with omega-6s. As the consumption of foods rich in omega-6s continues to stay high, obesity continues to climb. The following obesity statistics reveal the disturbing trends in Americans' health over the last two decades:[10]

- There are fifty-eight million overweight, forty million obese, and three million morbidly obese Americans
- Eight out of ten Americans over the age of twenty-five are overweight
- 78 percent of Americans are not meeting the basic recommended levels of daily exercises

- 25 percent of Americans are completely sedentary
- Since 1990 there has been a 76 percent increase in Type II diabetes among adults thirty to forty years old

Ironically, and most unfortunately, many of the very people who have been making an effort to eat healthier by substituting seed oils (such as corn, soy, safflower, and sesame) for animal fats have accumulated a lot more omega-6s in their bodies than they would have otherwise. Their metabolic rate has slowed down and as a result, they "could have a profound predisposition for obesity,"[11] says Professor Leonard Storlien at the University of Sydney in Australia. Professor Storlien, who studies the effect of dietary fats on obesity and insulin resistance, has found that "not only the quantity of dietary fat, but also the type of fat used, will produce different effects on body weight and metabolism."[12] In his experiments, foods rich in omega-3s can protect against obesity and diabetes. Another study, conducted by two Danish scientists, Dr. Jørn Dyerberg and Dr. Hans Olaf Bang, followed Eskimos of the Umanak district of Greenland, whose diet consists of fish, seal meat, and whale blubber. The scientists stated that despite very high saturated fat consumption, "not a single established case of diabetes mellitus is known at present in the population of the Umanak district."[13]

According to nutritional biochemist William E. M. Lands, a researcher at the National Institutes of Health and one of the world's foremost authorities on essential fatty acids, both omega-6s and omega-3s are competing for a certain enzyme in cell membranes called the desaturase enzyme. Although omega-3s are the preferred substrate of the enzyme, an excess of dietary omega-6s compared to omega-3s results in greater net formation of omega-6s.[14] Put more simply, if we consume too few omega-3s, the body will use an even smaller percent of those omega-3s, choosing the higher amount of omega-6s instead. All these new scientific discoveries point to one major conclusion: humans need to include plenty of omega-3s in their diet; otherwise their metabolism may slow down and they could start feeling sleepy and sluggish similar to a hibernating bear. As Dr. Burton Litman, a membrane biophysicist, concluded, "You couldn't be an astronaut or a fighter pilot if you were raised on an omega-3 deficient diet."[15]

So how can we achieve the healthiest balance of essential fatty acids? Most of the articles I read suggested that the ratio of omega-6s to omega-3s should be 3:1 or 2:1. The typical American diet today contains anywhere from a 10:1 to a 20:1 ratio of omega-6 to omega-3, an imbalance associated with a high rate of disease. The Institute of Medicine, the health arm of the National Academy of Sciences, recommends an intake of approximately 10:1, much higher than the ratio recommended by Sweden (5:1) or Japan (4:1). The ratio in Japan is associated with a very low incidence of heart and other disease.[16]

What can we do to increase our consumption of omega-3s? According to Dr. Frank Sacks, Professor of Nutrition at Harvard School of Public Health,[17] there are two major types of omega-3 fatty acids in our diets. One type is alpha-linolenic acid (ALA), which is found in flaxseed oil, walnuts, and also in green leafy vegetables. The other type, the longer-chain fatty acids eicosapentaenoic acid (EPA) and docosahexaenoic acid (DHA), is found in fatty fish. The body partially converts ALA to EPA and DHA.

Fortunately, omega-3 is widely available in all greens, especially in spinach, romaine lettuce, and arugula. One of the highest levels of omega-3 can be found in purslane, a widespread wild green. While several research papers stated that it was not certain if the parental molecule of omega-3 found in greens could be turned into DHA or EPA that the body could use, I was fortunate to find the following information: Dr. Ralph Holman, a biochemist who has focused his studies on lipids and fatty acids, researched the blood samples of thirty-eight Nigerians from Enugu, the capital city of Enugu State,

Nigeria. Dr. Holman found that the omega-3 content in this group was higher than in any population he had studied. These Nigerians didn't eat very much fish but they ate a lot of greens and had no omega-6-heavy vegetable oils in their diet.[18]

Other great sources of omega-3s are sprouted flax seed, sprouted chia seeds, and flaxseed oil. Flaxseed oil is the only fat allowed in the diets of cancer patients at the Gerson Institute in San Diego. Charlotte Gerson, the founder of the Gerson Institute, explained that according to their research, flaxseed oil is the only fat that does not promote the growth of cancer cells.[19] I now pour a tablespoon of flaxseed oil on my salads almost daily.

Omega-3s are very unstable and can become rancid extremely quickly, even inside our digestive tract. For example, flaxseed oil, which is highest in omega-3s, has to remain refrigerated; if it stays at room temperature even for twenty minutes it can become rancid. Ingesting rancid oil is dangerous because it can actually promote instead of prevent heart disease by forming lots of free radicals. To combat this problem, make sure to include a large variety of fresh fruit and vegetables in your meals that are rich in antioxidants, such as blueberries, blackberries, strawberries, raspberries, plums, oranges, grapes cherries, beets, red cabbage, colored bell peppers, kale, and others. The high-rancidity potential of omega-3 oils makes it difficult for manufacturers to produce, transport, and store oils such as flaxseed in mass quantity, which is why products rich in omega-3s are usually a lot more expensive. But I would rather pay for high-quality food now than for medical bills resulting from my poor nutrition later on.

Increasing the omega-3s in our diet is important but not enough; it is also crucial to decrease our consumption of omega-6s. "Fish consumption counts, but our problems are probably caused not by a lack of fish in our diets but by an overconsumption of seed oils and underconsumption of greens," writes Dr. Artemis Simopoulos in *The Omega Diet*.[20] This important information about essential fatty acids has helped me to find answers to some of the questions that I have been asking for years, such as why I and some other raw fooders gained extra weight on our diet and had a hard time losing it. The time has come for us all to carefully examine our diets and reduce or eliminate our intake of such oils as corn oil, sesame oil, safflower oil, sunflower oil, and peanut oil as well as reduce our consumption of nuts and seeds.

To help you make better dietary choices, using nutritional data from the USDA I have compiled the following list of ratios between omega-3s and omega-6s found in a variety of nuts, seeds, oils, greens, and fruit.[21]

I realize now that for a number of years I was fanatical about being a 100 percent raw foodist. I believed that anything raw was better than anything cooked. When I learned about the benefits of raw food, I didn't think twice—I was going to do it all the way. While in the beginning of my raw food diet (which consisted of fruits, vegetables, nuts, and seeds) I felt completely satisfied, several years later I started to feel that something was missing. I developed cravings that continued to grow stronger and more frequent until at last I felt constantly hungry. I enjoyed eating fruits and I could eat a pound or two of them in one sitting but after I was done, I was still hungry, which is a symptom of deficiency. Carrots, broccoli, and other such vegetables were not very appealing to me, especially when they were prepared with any kind of dressing made with oil. I had developed a strong dislike for any oils and after about ten years of being a raw foodist, I couldn't tolerate even a drop of oil in my food.

Ratio of Omega-3s to Omega-6s in Oils, Seeds, and Greens

Flaxseed oil: (1 tbsp)

Total Omega-3 fatty acids	7,196 mg (4.2 times more omega 3s)
Total Omega-6 fatty acids	715 mg

http://nutritiondata.self.com/facts/fats-and-oils/7554/2

Sunflower oil: (1 tbsp)

Total Omega-3 fatty acids	5.0 mg
Total Omega-6 fatty acids	3,905 mg (78 times more omega-6s)

http://nutritiondata.self.com/facts/fats-and-oils/7945/2

Safflower oil: (1 tbsp)

Total Omega-3 fatty acids	0 mg
Total Omega-6 fatty acids	10,073 mg (too much! omega-6s)

http://nutritiondata.self.com/facts/fats-and-oils/573/2

Sesame oil: (1 tbsp)

Total Omega-3 fatty acids	40.5 mg
Total Omega-6 fatty acids	5,576 mg (1,138 times more omega-6s)

http://nutritiondata.self.com/facts/fats-and-oils/511/2

Corn oil: (1 tbsp)

Total Omega-3 fatty acids	157 mg
Total Omega-6 fatty acids	7,224 mg (46 times more omega-6s)

http://nutritiondata.self.com/facts/fats-and-oils/580/2

Canola oil: (1 tbsp)

Total Omega-3 fatty acids	1,031 mg
Total Omega-6 fatty acids	2,532 mg (2.5 times more omega-6s)

http://nutritiondata.self.com/facts/fats-and-oils/7947/2

Olive oil: (1 tbsp)

Total Omega-3 fatty acids	103 mg
Total Omega-6 fatty acids	1,318 mg (13 times more omega-6s)

http://nutritiondata.self.com/facts/fats-and-oils/509/2

Ratio of Omega-3s to Omega-6s in Oils, Seeds, and Greens

Chia seeds: (1 ounce)

Total Omega-3 fatty acids	4,915 mg (3 times more omega-3s)
Total Omega-6 fatty acids	1,620 mg

http://nutritiondata.self.com/facts/nut-and-seed-products/3061/2

Flax seeds: (1 ounce)

Total Omega-3 fatty acids	6,388 mg (3.9 times more omega-3s)
Total Omega-6 fatty acids	1,655 mg

http://nutritiondata.self.com/facts/nut-and-seed-products/3163/2

Sunflower seeds: (1 cup)

Total Omega-3 fatty acids	34.0 mg
Total Omega-6 fatty acids	10,602 mg (312 times more omega-6s)

http://nutritiondata.self.com/facts/nut-and-seed-products/3076/2

Sesame seeds: (1 cup)

Total Omega-3 fatty acids	541 mg
Total Omega-6 fatty acids	30,776 mg (57 times more omega-6s)

http://nutritiondata.self.com/facts/nut-and-seed-products/3070/2

Pumpkin seeds: (1 cup)

Total Omega-3 fatty acids	250 mg
Total Omega-6 fatty acids	28,571 mg (114 times more omega-6s)

http://nutritiondata.self.com/facts/nut-and-seed-products/3066/2

Walnuts: (1 cup)

Total Omega-3 fatty acids	10,623 mg
Total Omega-6 fatty acids	44,567 mg (4.2 times more omega-6s)

http://nutritiondata.self.com/facts/nut-and-seed-products/3138/2

Almonds: (1 cup)

Total Omega-3 fatty acids	5.7 mg
Total Omega-6 fatty acids	11,462 mg (2,000 times more omega-6s)

http://nutritiondata.self.com/facts/nut-and-seed-products/3085/2

Ratio of Omega-3s to Omega-6s in Oils, Seeds, and Greens

Pecans: (1 cup)

Total Omega-3 fatty acids	1,075 mg
Total Omega-6 fatty acids	22,487 mg (21 times more omega-6s)

http://nutritiondata.self.com/facts/nut-and-seed-products/3129/2

Wheat: (1 cup)

Total Omega-3 fatty acids	52 mg
Total Omega-6 fatty acids	1,152 mg (22 times more omega-6s)

http://nutritiondata.self.com/facts/cereal-grains-and-pasta/5737/2

Rye: (1 cup)

Total Omega-3 fatty acids	265. mg
Total Omega-6 fatty acids	1,619 mg (6 times more omega-6s)

http://nutritiondata.self.com/facts/cereal-grains-and-pasta/5727/2

Oats: (1 cup)

Total Omega-3 fatty acids	173. mg
Total Omega-6 fatty acids	3,781 mg (22 times more omega-6s)

http://nutritiondata.self.com/facts/cereal-grains-and-pasta/5708/2

Quinoa: (1 cup)

Total Omega-3 fatty acids	522 mg
Total Omega-6 fatty acids	5,061 mg (10 times more omega-6s)

http://nutritiondata.self.com/facts/cereal-grains-and-pasta/5705/2

Lentils: (1 cup)

Total Omega-3 fatty acids	209 mg
Total Omega-6 fatty acids	776 mg (3.7 times more omega-6s)

http://nutritiondata.self.com/facts/legumes-and-legume-products/4337/2

Beans, snap, green, raw: (1 cup)

Total Omega-3 fatty acids	39.6. mg (1.6 times more omega-3s)
Total Omega-6 fatty acids	25.3 mg

http://nutritiondata.self.com/facts/vegetables-and-vegetable-products/2341/2

Ratio of Omega-3s to Omega-6s in Oils, Seeds, and Greens

Chickpeas, raw: (1 cup)

Total Omega-3 fatty acids	202 mg
Total Omega-6 fatty acids	5,186 mg (26 times more omega-6s)

http://nutritiondata.self.com/facts/legumes-and-legume-products/4325/2

Green Peas, raw: (1 cup)

Total Omega-3 fatty acids	50.8 mg
Total Omega-6 fatty acids	220 mg (4.3 times more omega-6s)

http://nutritiondata.self.com/facts/vegetables-and-vegetable-products/2520/2

Sugar snap peas, raw: (1 cup)

Total Omega-3 fatty acids	12.7 mg
Total Omega-6 fatty acids7	3.5 mg (5.8 times more omega-6s)

http://nutritiondata.self.com/facts/vegetables-and-vegetable-products/2516/2

Lettuce, green leaf, raw: (1 head, 360 g)

Total Omega-3 fatty acids	209 mg (2.4 times more omega-3s)
Total Omega-6 fatty acids	86.4 mg

http://nutritiondata.self.com/facts/vegetables-and-vegetable-products/2477/2

Lettuce, cos or romaine, raw: (1 head, 626 g)

Total Omega-3 fatty acids	707 mg (2.4 times more omega-3s)
Total Omega-6 fatty acids	294 mg

http://nutritiondata.self.com/facts/vegetables-and-vegetable-products/2475/2

Spinach, raw: (1 bunch, 340 g)

Total Omega-3 fatty acids	469 mg (5.3 times more omega-3s)
Total Omega-6 fatty acids	88.4 mg

http://nutritiondata.self.com/facts/vegetables-and-vegetable-products/2626/2

Ratio of Omega-3s to Omega-6s in Oils, Seeds, and Greens

Dandelion greens, raw: (100 g)

Total Omega-3 fatty acids	44 mg
Total Omega-6 fatty acids	261 mg (5.9 times more omega-6s)

http://nutritiondata.self.com/facts/vegetables-and-vegetable-products/2441/2

Arugula, raw: (100 g)

Total Omega-3 fatty acids	170 mg (1.3 times more omega-3s)
Total Omega-6 fatty acids	130 mg

http://nutritiondata.self.com/facts/vegetables-and-vegetable-products/3025/2

Apples, raw: (1 medium size)

Total Omega-3 fatty acids	16.4 mg
Total Omega-6 fatty acids	78.3 mg (4.8 times more omega-6s)

http://nutritiondata.self.com/facts/fruits-and-fruit-juices/1809/2

Bananas, raw: (1 medium size)

Total Omega-3 fatty acids	31.9 mg
Total Omega-6 fatty acids	54.3 mg (1.7 times more omega-6s)

http://nutritiondata.self.com/facts/fruits-and-fruit-juices/1846/2

Strawberries, raw: (100 g)

Total Omega-3 fatty acids	65.0 mg
Total Omega-6 fatty acids	90.0 mg (1.4 times more omega-6s)

http://nutritiondata.self.com/facts/fruits-and-fruit-juices/2064/2

Carrots, raw: (100 g)

Total Omega-3 fatty acids	2.0 mg
Total Omega-6 fatty acids	115 mg (57 times more omega-6s)

http://nutritiondata.self.com/facts/vegetables-and-vegetable-products/2383/2

Unfortunately, my solution to satisfy my cravings while staying on a 100 percent raw food diet was to increase my consumption of seeds and nuts. In the late '90s, several companies in the United States began manufacturing new lines of health products, including organic raw tahini (ground sesame seeds) and a number of raw organic nut butters such as almond, cashew, and pumpkin, designed especially for raw foodists. One of these manufactures was located in our home of Ashland, Oregon. I started to buy nut butters on a regular basis and even ordered in bulk, buying a case at a time. At first, eating more nuts and nut butters seemed to help me with my cravings and I thought that I had found the solution to my problems. However, after several months of consuming too many nuts, I noticed that my health had begun to decline. My energy went down, my nails became brittle, and I developed several cavities in my teeth. Worst of all, I started gaining weight. It wasn't until I came up with the idea of green smoothies in 2004 and began drinking them daily that I experienced a profound improvement in my health and lost some weight. I understand now that I had added the necessary omega-3s to my diet but still had not reduced the omega-6s.

I continued consuming nuts on a regular basis, as I thought them to be a necessary source of good fat for raw vegans but to my surprise, I was becoming less and less fond of nuts. To continue consuming them, I started preparing "gourmet nuts," enhancing their taste with different herbs and fruits. I became really good at making these delicious mixtures, but despite my efforts, the time came when I was not able to consume any nuts or seeds at all. If I ate any amount of nuts, I instantly developed a sore throat and fever that would last several hours. A few times I visited potlucks in different raw food communities and accidentally consumed nuts without being aware that I had done so. Each time nuts had the same effect on me and I had to leave the party.

At one of my lectures in St. Petersburg, Russia, a young man told me an interesting story. As an experiment, he once ate nothing but nuts and seeds for six months. His rationale was that if people could live on fast food, he should be able to live on raw organic nuts and seeds. After six months he passed out on the street and was taken to an emergency room, diagnosed with brain seizures. When he explained to doctors about his experiment, the doctors told him never to eat nuts or seeds again.

For a long time I couldn't find an explanation for my body's rejection of nuts and didn't know what to do about my diet until I read the very latest research about the dangers of overconsumption of omega-6 fatty acids that could cause a deficiency of omega-3 fatty acids.

While I still consider a raw diet to be optimal, I don't want to fanatically follow a 100 percent raw food diet at the expense of my health. When asked, I respond that my diet now is about 95 percent raw. If I had to choose between raw nuts and steamed vegetables, I would go for steamed vegetables. As I continue my life and my research, my diet might slightly change again.

I find it remarkable that the highest concentrations of alpha-linolenic acid, the parent omega-3 fat, are found in the chloroplasts of green leaves, where it assists plants with their most active process, photosynthesis, the basis of all life on earth.[22] Because the available nutritional data shows that greens are the second highest vegetarian source of omega-3s after flaxseed oil, they are very clearly important for helping us get enough essential omega-3 fatty acids in our diet. Considering all the benefits that we can get from omega-3s, green smoothies are simply a miraculous healing drink. I enjoy my green smoothies every day. I prefer to associate myself with a humming-bird rather than with a hibernating bear.

A Tribute to Dr. Ann

I truly admire Dr. Ann Wigmore. Whenever I order a shot of wheatgrass, I feel like I personally know Dr. Ann. Wheatgrass juice makes me healthier. I owe the opportunity of drinking it at my local co-op to Dr. Ann. Thanks to her, people around the world can drink wheatgrass juice and enjoy its countless healing benefits. I find it amazing how Ann Wigmore is continuing to touch our lives decades after she passed away, even though many of us have never met her or even heard her name.

Not only did Dr. Ann discover and thoroughly research the great healing properties of wheatgrass, she also developed and thoroughly described the process of growing wheatgrass in trays at home or any location. She came up with an inexpensive wheatgrass juicer to make this elixir of life available to everyone.

I appreciate many of Dr. Ann's inventions, which we all conveniently utilize in our everyday lives while thinking that they have existed forever. Who today remembers that raw gourmet food began with Dr. Ann's "seed cheese" and "raw soup" recipes? She invented nut milks, dehydrated crackers, almond loaf, and "live" candy for us.

Dr. Ann introduced a variety of sprouts into our lives. She also came up with a sprouting bag. Whenever my family travels, we always pack sprouting seeds to guarantee a fresh supply of greens. Dr. Ann called sprouts "living foods." It is hard to imagine that these words didn't exist some time ago.

Dr. Ann discovered the many healing benefits of blending foods, especially greens. She lived the last several years of her life almost completely on blended foods, a large part of which consisted of greens. She noticed that blended foods assimilated into her system more easily. For instance, she would say about fruit, "If I have an apple, I will blend it instead of munch it, because I don't want to waste its energy or mine." She observed that eating blended food gave her superior health and cut her hours of sleep down to two hours per night.[1]

Before Dr. Ann, people utilized blenders for "insignificant" purposes like whipping eggs and making cocktails. Today, we cannot imagine a raw food kitchen without a powerful blender.

Dr. Ann clearly saw the tight connection between organic soil and human health, and she began promoting organic gardening and composting in the 1960s when most people were just beginning to embrace chemical fertilizers as the future of agriculture.

I see Ann Wigmore's uniqueness in her ability to pay attention to a wide spectrum of events, to explore living on this planet as one whole process, and to apply her expertise to many different aspects of life. She didn't choose to be a specialist in just one narrow field, as many others have done. She dared to form her personal opinion about everything she encountered, be it blood analysis, colonic irrigations, fasting, food composition, bacteria, gardening, or drinking water. Due to her all-inclusive vision, she was able to create a healing system that has helped thousands of people.

Dr. Ann was known to work vigorously and productively. She invented new ideas daily. She kept herself in notably excellent shape, always running, never walking, sustaining herself on just two hours of sleep per day. At the ripe age of eighty-two, Dr. Ann didn't have a single gray hair. This fact was so unbelievable that her students asked her permission to study her hair in a lab to see if it was dyed. The test proved that it was her natural color.

In addition to her profound research in the field of human health, Dr. Ann was an animal rights activist, fought against the fluoridation and chlorination of drinking water, and was against chemical pollution and many other things.

The latest discoveries in science prove Dr. Ann was right in the majority of her predictions and recommendations. I believe the day will come when medical students will study Ann Wigmore's books as they study Hippocrates today.

Dr. Ann is well recognized all around the world. In my travels I continue to encounter people who ask me if I have heard of Dr. Ann Wigmore. This inquiry is usually followed by an exciting story about another human life saved by Dr. Ann's teachings. I doubt it is possible to calculate just how many lives this brilliant woman has saved. She herself was one of the healthiest people on the planet in the twentieth century. Dr. Ann was living her talk and practicing in her own life everything that she was teaching. Most of all, however, people who met her in person remember her for her benevolent, loving spirit.

Testimonials

LOST 120 POUNDS AND HEALED MULTIPLE CHRONIC ILLNESSES

I am a thirty-seven-year-old woman. Three years ago I weighed 250 pounds and I was very sick all the time. I ate fast food three times a day, guzzled Pepsi all the time, and smoked cigarettes. I never ate fresh fruit or vegetables, and I had no idea how badly I was hurting my body. I suffered from many afflictions: I had severe depression that I had been treating with antidepressants for ten years. I had chronic allergies, chronic bronchitis, chronic bladder infections, arthritis, headaches, horrible menstrual cramps, muscle aches, irritable bowel syndrome, stomach cramps, lethargy, and I'm sure there is more that I can't even remember right now. I had my gallbladder removed, and I was sure once it was removed that I would start feeling better. Instead, the opposite happened. I immediately went right back to fast food and Pepsi, and I continued to become sicker. I felt much worse after the surgery; I didn't know what to do, and

I was sure that if I did not figure something out soon that I was going to die.

I started researching food and quickly realized that I had been poisoning my body for thirty-four years. I started eating fewer processed foods with less fat. I felt somewhat better, but I didn't feel great. Soon I came across some raw food books, and after about six months of struggling with food addictions I went entirely raw. I lost 120 pounds, and I felt really good for about a year. After a year of eating raw I started gaining weight, feeling tired all the time, and having horrible stomach pain just like I used to. About that time I read *Green for Life*. I realized through this book that I was still consuming too much fat and not enough greens. So I started drinking green smoothies. I immediately felt fantastic—better than I'd ever felt before. I continue to feel great today, and I drink green smoothies all the time. Thank you, Victoria, for your wonderful book and insight.

—*Victoria Everett*

ROSACEA DISAPPEARS

My boyfriend and I began drinking green smoothies in November 2009 after reading your wonderful book *Green for Life*. Almost instantly we felt more energetic, lost cravings for sweets and junk food, and dropped about ten pounds each. My boyfriend grew up with problem skin—acne and rosacea. He has tried *everything*— prescription medications, over-the-counter topical treatments, Proactiv, and nothing ever worked. When I began the smoothies, the green color scared him a bit, but then I doctored them and made them really sweet and purple or pink rather than green, and he was hooked. His skin has never looked better. His face is no longer red from rosacea, and he no longer breaks out with pimples. And we *know* it's from the smoothies because if we go away and he doesn't drink the smoothies for a day or two, out come the pimples. I don't have skin issues, but my hair was thinning and it would never grow long. My nails were also brittle and weak and would not grow. Now after my own "smoothie revolution," my hair is all the way down my back, my nails are strong and I get them manicured weekly, and I feel fantastic! Now we are on a mission to eat mostly organic, cut out all high-fructose corn syrup and processed foods, and be as chemical-free as possible. This is all because of you, Victoria, and your wonderful book. We bought a Blendtec blender for Christmas 2008, and it has been the greatest investment in our health. Thank you again for bringing this amazing concept into our lives. We will keep up with the daily smoothies and other healthy and "clean" ways of eating to lose weight and for me to finally come off my blood pressure medications. I have been taken off my cholesterol medications, so I am halfway there!

—*Jenny Rogers, New York City*

CRAVINGS FOR COOKED FOOD DISAPPEARED

I have tried for several years—unsuccessfully—to switch to the raw food diet. Although I love how I feel when eating raw foods, cravings for cooked foods usually get in the way. Eventually I am back on cooked foods completely.

Although I was on a vegan diet, I still ate mostly cooked and processed foods. My health began to deteriorate. I had regular heart palpitations and kidney pain; I was tired, grumpy, and lazy; I couldn't think clearly and had very poor memory; my skin looked a bit gray and unhealthy; I had swelling in my legs; my arms and legs were very sensitive to touch, and if I bumped into anything I would be in extreme pain. Recently I began drinking one glass of green smoothie a day. (I've read all your books and love them, by the way). One day when feeling particularly bad I decided that I would add another green smoothie each day so I would have two glasses instead of my usual one.

Well, the funniest thing happened. When I added the second glass, on the very first day I began to get extreme cravings for certain live foods. For example, I suddenly craved cucumber, and I ran to the store to buy some. Then when I finished with my cucumber craving, I wanted tomatoes. I blended half a Vita-Mix full of tomato juice and drank it down. This continued with different greens and vegetables for a few days. But instead of going back to my old way of eating, I kept craving raw foods. It has been a month now with no cravings for cooked foods. For the past several days I've been drawn to green juices and have several glasses a day. I feel fantastic. I have lots of energy, I feel happier, the swelling in my legs went away, my heart palpitations have stopped, my kidney pain went away, my memory is better, my thoughts are clearer, and I even noticed that my hearing improved; I didn't even know it was bad before that.

My husband and I are both eating raw foods now with plenty of greens, either in a smoothie, which we have every day, or in salads.

Thank you so much for all your efforts to help the rest of us find the way to health! You are an amazing and inspiring family.

—*Raja, San Diego*

GOT OFF MEDICATIONS
FOR ANXIETY AND ALLERGIES

I purchased the book *12 Steps to Raw Foods,* and I had a hard time putting the book down after starting. What I love about the book are the truths that all of our "normal everyday foods" were full of toxic poisons from pesticides and chemicals. My personal trainer had tried to tell me some of the bad chemicals and such that were in foods, but I shrugged it off—I guess sometimes it takes reading a good book to make a person wake up and stop fighting the idea. After all, what do you have to lose? In the past I was the girl who could eat all the junk I could find and stay skinny and peppy. Well, now that I am thirty-three, things have changed. I was sick of being moody, sick of not feeling "good." I was on medication for anxiety and seasonal allergies; now I have stopped taking the meds. Although I feel I have a ways to go, I know that I have a wonderful path to follow now on my way to a healthier, happier me.

I have been making a combo smoothie of fruits and greens for over two months now. I am up to half fruit and half greens. I have seen a difference in my energy levels, my mood swings are much better, and I even tend to crave healthy raw foods that I didn't quite care for in the past. I love the book and the ideas to help get me to a better, healthier life. Reading about raw foods has also brought new conversation to the dinner table and social outings. Thank you!

—*Mandy W.*

LIFELONG SORE HEALED

When J. C. came to visit me four years ago in New Mexico, he wanted to put kale in my smoothies. It sounded disgusting to me. He finally convinced me to try it at least once. He put an entire huge bunch of kale in the blender. I ignored the color, drank it, and realized that it was actually not bad. At that time I had a sore on my hand about the size of a quarter that would not heal. It was the spot where a lump had been removed by a doctor in Sweden when I lived there. That doctor told me to get used to the raw spot on my hand; she said I would probably have it for life. This raw spot was painful to the touch, and it hurt to even have fabric brush against it. J. C. visited me for months. We had green smoothies each day. I noticed that within a few weeks my hand was beginning to heal, and within three months the painful spot on my hand healed completely. I now live with J. C., and I am the queen of our morning smoothies. They have gone from banana-rich sweet smoothies to many more greens and much less sweet fruits. Our tastes have changed, and our smoothies are our favorite meal of the day. We feel great!

—*Rae Sikora*

PEACEFUL, NATURAL CHILDBIRTH

My first labor and delivery was very difficult: twenty-four-plus hours of agony and full of complications. I am one of those moms who would have died in childbirth fifty years ago. I react badly to the hormones produced by the body at the onset of labor; symptoms appear suddenly and are quite serious—no platelets (no ability to clot blood), liver and kidney failure, and seizures. They couldn't give me a C-section because I wouldn't have survived the surgery. It was truly a miracle that my son finally got out and we both survived.

For my second pregnancy a year later, I had discovered raw food, self-hypnosis, and was a devotee of the green smoothie. I was mostly raw and vegan, but not a hundred percent; I drank about one quart of green smoothie per day. Although my doctor and midwife were very anxious about my low protein intake, I had an easy pregnancy and gave birth to my eleven-pound Ivan in less than two hours with no drugs and almost pain-free. I happened to lose over a quart of blood during this process because he was so big, but I felt just fine and recovered pretty quickly. During my pregnancy, as with many women, I was extremely sensitive to smell, taste, chemicals, etc. What I particularly noticed about green smoothies, even though they are fairly bitter, was that they were always calming to my stomach and my nerves. They made me full without bloating and without digestive issues; they kept my digestion moving very reliably and comfortably. My diet and especially green smoothies are what enabled me to have a peaceful natural birthing for my second child. Thanks, Victoria!

—*Rosanna D'Agnillo, Carmichael, California*

SINUS INFECTION DISAPPEARS— BODY REJUVENATES

Over the past few years I have experienced a lot of stress in my life. Over time it certainly takes its toll on a person's body. I have been seeing a nutritionist/chiropractor for almost a year now. The supplements he has prescribed have definitely helped me, but still I continued to pick up almost every bug that came along, felt run down, had difficulty sleeping, and so on. I was exercising but had to force myself to do so. It seemed that I would stay well for two or three weeks at the most before I would fall prey to another virus or bacteria of some sort. The nutritionist kept telling me that my adrenal glands were worn out.

During the summer a friend told me about her green smoothie lifestyle, and though I briefly considered trying it, I did not pursue it. Then at the end of November 2009 I got yet another bug. I was so tired and frustrated by then that I went to see the nutritionist three times in two weeks trying to get relief from my symptoms. Instead I began reacting to the supplements that I was taking. One night I was lying on the living room sofa at 2 a.m., trying not to cough my head off and wake up the rest of the household. I began praying fervently that God would give me an answer and bring healing into my body. In a series of events that I believe to be God-orchestrated, a couple of days later I was reading a book called *Toxic Relief* by Dr. Don Colbert and I sensed that God was telling me to make a drastic change to my diet. I recalled my friend's testimony about green smoothies, and I began doing research. Fortunately, my husband was agreeable to the whole change, and the next day I ordered my Vita-Mix. As soon as it arrived we began drinking smoothies made from organic produce. Overnight I could sense a big difference in the sinus infection that I had been fighting. In a few days I could feel a difference in my energy level, and I was falling asleep more easily, waking earlier, and feeling more rested. My sinuses were like a faucet, however. So I went back to the nutritionist, thinking I had yet another bug of some sort.

He began his usual process of muscle-testing me, and he looked at me in stunned amazement. I was testing as "strong" for the first time ever. He said he believed the mucus draining was part of my detoxification process and not to worry about it, and he took me off of almost all of the supplements that I had been taking. He said that as long as I was drinking the green smoothies, I was doing the best thing for my body that I could possibly do. A couple of days later the drainage cleared up. I was feeling so much better that I began exercising in earnest. In addition to working out at a fitness center, I joined a couple of friends at a weekly Pilates class. The first week of the Pilates class, the instructor had us moving in ways that my body may never have moved. I expected to be really sore afterward, but I was not—in fact, I have been exercising quite a bit and have almost no stiffness or soreness whatsoever. It is totally amazing. Thank you for your research and your books.

—*Vicki Cramer, Escondido, Calif.*

BOWEL SURGERY AVOIDED

I have eaten one hundred percent raw food for one year—November 2008 to December 2009. I had been having diverticulitis attacks every three months for four years. I was so worried about my future because I was shitting the bed at night and not even realizing it until it was too late. I also had severe gas problems that smelled horrible. When I started raw, I had severe diarrhea for a month, but I hung in there with support from my naturopath because I was willing to try anything. Doctors wanted to remove a section of my bowel, and I was almost ready for them to do it. Things gradually changed with my green smoothies. I have not had any bowel-control problems now for a year and no attacks at all. I have to be careful to stay away from vegetables that I am allergic to like Swiss chard. I do eat fish now and some cooked vegetables because my thyroid function is low, and greens like broccoli and kale have something in them that is hard on the thyroid when they are eaten raw. I gained weight while I was eating a hundred percent raw, so I'm just experimenting now to find my body's balance. I will never give up my green smoothies, which I share with my husband in the mornings.

—*Carollyne Kaise, Toronto*

MY YEAR OF GREEN SMOOTHIES

I started drinking green smoothies in January 2009 after reading some raw food sites on the Internet. During 2007 and 2008 I had gained about twenty-six pounds after I returned to work as a teacher, along with the emotional impact of my mother's death. I felt lethargic and had low energy, severe upper-back and neck muscle tension, and anxiety, and I had a decreasing interest in work and life. I was also having cravings for sugar, coffee, chocolate, and chips. My gallstone symptoms had worsened, with pain in my shoulder and neck, headaches with nausea, vomiting, bloating, stomach pain, and severe tiredness, so I had to start taking over-the-counter pain killers again.

Before my diagnosis in 1995 of a malignant right temporal lobe glioma brain tumor, I thought I was a very healthy eater—an on-and-off vegetarian since age twelve who ate no sugar or processed fast food, had no weight issues, was a nonsmoker and nondrinker, and didn't take any type of medicine at all. When I was diagnosed, mainstream medicine took over my life. I felt all my choices being taken away, and I became a patient. My illness continued for the next nine years until 2004, when I took control of my own health after nearly dying from a grand mal seizure caused by low sodium from epilepsy medication and poor nutrition. My fifteen-year-old daughter hadn't gone to school that day and basically saved my life by calling an ambulance. I had stopped breathing, and my lungs had collapsed. I was unaware of anything until I woke up in intensive care three days later, intubated.

When I returned home after a week, I decided to stop taking all the prescription medications they had sent me home with—

no more prescription narcotic painkillers like oxycodone and MS Contin, Valium, over-the-counter painkillers, "just in case" epilepsy medications, or antinausea tablets. These had all severely affected my quality of life and nervous system for nine years to the point that I could not work, get out of bed, or leave home for days at my lowest point. In hindsight I had undiagnosed significant depression resulting from my cancer and treatment, and the painkillers were masking/numbing this.

I started feeling better within a week, and what had been like a massive black fog lifted out of my brain. I was back in my body, and I gradually got out of bed. Interestingly, my sense of taste and smell came back. During a detox that seemed to last more than a year, I decided to research nutrition and start eating a more nutritious diet, which I have been doing for the last four years. As I started researching nutrition my first priority was finding out about sodium. I then compiled a list of all the foods that appeared most frequently and were highest on all the vitamin and mineral lists. I decided to start eating more of these foods and building my diet around them. I ate them cooked because I only have one molar on my bottom jaw due to damage from radiotherapy and medications so I cannot chew food very well, especially raw food. The food and nutrients we consume are so underrated and ignored by the medical profession—nutrition is not studied comprehensively in medical school and I have had years of dealing with doctors whose only treatment or way of thinking is reaching for the prescription pad.

Before discovering green smoothies, I thought I was eating a healthy diet that suited my up-and-down blood sugar levels, hormonal problems (early menopause at thirty-six) and low sodium caused by radiotherapy. My usual diet was porridge (cooked rolled oats and barley with dried fruit, raw apple and seeds with rice milk) cooked vegetables, mainly soups using lots of pumpkin sweet potato /nuts/seeds/beans/tofu/fish/whole grains. I ate no dairy, wheat, or meat except fish and no processed food, but I was eating no fresh raw food at all and very few greens. I somehow knew that eating more live raw food would be the answer, but my main obstacle to eating more live food was my teeth.

After I discovered green smoothies—drinking about two quarts a day, half for breakfast and the rest in the afternoon—within a few days to a week I felt the difference in my digestion, bloating, and energy levels. I had fewer cravings and blood sugar ups and downs. I had stable mood levels throughout the day, more motivation and concentration, fewer gallstone symptoms, and immediate weight loss. My skin feels better and my teeth are whiter. I felt motivated enough to get back to regular exercise and yoga. I have also stopped drinking coffee and even wanting tea; I used to put honey in my tea (no milk), but have no desire at all for sweet things or caffeine. My only craving now is for fresh raw food—green smoothies!

Other differences I have noticed are that my nails are stronger, my skin feels much less dry, and my eyes are definitely brighter—and greener! The main thing is that I feel something I can only describe as "zingier," like an internal buzzy feeling of something that just feels right. My increased energy and exercise mean no more muscle tension and joint pain and no visits to the chiropractor. I feel that my mind and body are generally more in balance. There has been an amazing ripple effect: I have lost the extra twenty-six pounds and am maintaining my weight at 132 pounds without even having to think about it. In the last year of drinking green smoothies, I have not needed to take any over-the-counter pain relief or reflux and antacid medicines.

Since buying Victoria's green smoothie book last year, I have simplified my recipe and now use more of just one or two greens (3–5 cups) with some fruit and water. I have noticed that as my sweetness cravings have diminished, I no longer use bananas and sometimes use just an apple. The most exciting thing is exploring all the organic greens that are being grown locally and sold at the farmer's markets or the organic shops. Initially I used the more available spinach, baby spinach, English spinach, bok choy, choy sum (previously would have only cooked these), silverbeet (chard), cos lettuce (romaine) celery, cucumber, and flat-leaf parsley. Then I discovered this whole other world of greens: purslane, watercress, dandelion greens, chicory, sorrel, carrot and beetroot tops, endive, mizuna, tatsoi, and different types of dark green and red lettuce. When I discover a green for the first time, I salivate and cannot wait to get it home to blend.

There was a period in the middle of the year when I was spending too much money on all the organic fruit and vegetables, so I went back to cooked food. Within a few days I felt the difference: lethargy, bloating, constipation, aching joints and muscles, and zero energy. So I went back to green smoothies and a commitment to them for life. When I visit family and eat cooked and over-salted food, I immediately have a return of gallstone symptoms to the extent that I have to spend the next day on rice cakes and water before returning to green smoothies and raw food. I had to buy a blender to leave at my family's home for my next visits!

I think it's wonderful that something so simple and easy as a green smoothie can have such a positive impact in your life; it's also cheap and can be made with a minimum of equipment and effort. It is really easy to fit into people's busy, crazy, pressured lives. I am so inspired with how great I feel that I want to give everyone I know green smoothie recipes and demos and to try and inspire them too. My son recently bought his own blender for smoothies and is drinking over a quart a day. We have interesting arguments and discussions on nutrition; he has just finished a bachelor's in medical science and had believed that a meal wasn't worth eating unless it was meat-based. He can't believe how filling green smoothies are considering they are only greens and fruits.

My twenty-year-old daughter drank over a quart of smoothie every day when she was staying with me over Christmas (specially made for a beginner—2 cups baby spinach or spinach and mango or frozen watermelon, banana, and ginger). She loved it. She read your green smoothie book while she was here and took my copy home with her. The next day she texted me to say that she was convinced—and she was green smoothie ingredient shopping, asking for my advice. She doesn't like her smoothies too sweet either now and is adding more greens. My children and I e-mail or talk daily about what we've used in our green smoothies!

—N. A.

HEALED FROM A STROKE IN TWENTY-FOUR HOURS

Bagels and fragels and coffee, oh, my!

Despite the glowing health, weight loss, and incredible calm I had felt during Victoria's Joy for Life retreat, within two months I was eating large amounts of animal fat, meat, pasta, coffee drinks, bagels, and ice cream. If it didn't have salt, sugar, and dairy products in it, you probably wouldn't find it on my plate. The exception was green smoothies—I loved my smoothies and continued drinking one to two quarts a day after the retreat.

On Memorial Day I woke up at 4 a.m. and felt weird as heck. My left arm and left leg just weren't working right. I staggered to the bathroom, chewed a couple of aspirin, and crawled into bed. By the next day my speech had returned. I got to my doctor's office before anyone was there and sat on his front porch. When he arrived he walked up to me and said, "Why are you leaning to the left?" He sent me over to the hospital for testing. In a little over twenty-four hours I had recovered 90 percent of my functionality and strength. I went through all the tests, which all came back negative. Their conclusion was that due to obesity and hypertension I had suffered a stroke, but because of green smoothies they couldn't find any medical traces of the stroke, and I had recovered unbelievably quickly. What my doctor told me was that poor eating had caused my obesity and cardiac issues, and that superb nutrition had saved me.

I still struggle with the siren call of the SAD (standard American diet), but I never struggle with my green smoothies. It is what keeps me out of hospital and in a happy productive life. I've lost twenty pounds and plan on losing another sixty-five. My favorite smoothie depends on what season it is: in summer, kale and watermelon; in fall, parsley, apples, and cinnamon; in winter, spinach and pineapple; and in spring, dandelions and mangoes.

There are days when I wish I could just fix a glass of delicious green stuff for everyone on the planet. Childhood obesity is at epidemic proportions in the United States along with heart disease and cancer. The answer is simple and easily within our grasp.

—*Kate, Ann Arbor, Michigan*

GOT OFF BREATHING MACHINE

I started the raw journey one year ago this February. One of the first books I read was *Green for Life*. Since reading it and starting to drink green smoothies every day, I have lost over forty pounds and have stopped using a breathing machine at night. Getting dairy out of my diet was the key. I have been a vegetarian for twenty years but was still not as healthy as I am today. I still ate dairy, processed meat substitutes, and other processed vegetarian foods. Now I am 80 to 90 percent raw!

I drink a full Vita-Mix blender of green smoothie every day. I look younger, feel better, and am sleeping wonderfully. I really feel that green smoothies are the answer to so many medical conditions that people suffer from. I wish everyone would drink them.

My husband and I have taken classes at the Living Light Culinary Art Institute in Fort Bragg, California, to achieve our Raw Food Nutrition Educator certification, taught by doctors Rick and Karen

Dina. We are now spreading the word of green smoothies and raw food. It is our dream that everyone will experience the wonderful and miraculous benefits of living food, especially green smoothies.

—*Jeanne Westphal, Crescent City, California*

MYSTERY SKIN CONDITION HEALED

I thought you might like to hear about my daughter, Molly. She is the real reason that I started on green smoothies. She has been battling a mystery skin problem for two and a half years that started in her ear after swimming in a lake. I started treating her naturally for a fungal problem, but then went to a regular MD, who tested it and said it was staph. At this point it was so bad and so close to her brain that I said OK to antibiotics. This turned out like I figured it would: they did no good, and actually made her condition worse. I then decided to go with the gut approach; as long as she stayed off sugar and dairy and took all her nutrients, it was better, but never went away for good. Then it got really bad again, so in October I took her to a nutrition-minded MD. He said he didn't think it was staph and thought it was a gut issue as well. Once again she didn't stay on her protocol because it wasn't making that much difference.

My sister-in-law asked Molly if she would try green smoothies for a month and lent me your book; Molly and I started smoothies on December 14. I then ordered your latest book, and we are trying the different recipes. After just one month, her skin looks, as she said, "almost like a normal person's." It looks the best it has since her symptoms started two and a half years ago, and this is what is most amazing: I found an empty Little Debbie box in her room along with a receipt from Arby's for mozzarella sticks and a milk shake, not to mention all the Christmas sweets she must have eaten. She is leaving today for a youth retreat, and she asked me to make smoothies to take with her.

Thanks for all your research and information. I have known all along that we didn't eat enough veggies, but now we can, even if the rest of the family doesn't want to have them. I'm looking forward to my health improving also as I have bad adrenal issues and have to take forty nutrient pills a day—and I have actually already stopped taking my potassium and zinc.

—*Missy Hester*

HEALED HYPOGLYCEMIA, ARTHRITIS, AND CONSTIPATION

I have read all of your books and am grateful for the information you are so kindly offering to the world. I was so tired of just eating. My diet was healthy cooked foods, but I had to eat a lot of meat due to my hypoglycemia. I hated my diet as I was not allowed to eat any fruit. I ate that way for nine years, and I was overweight and could not lose one pound. I aged drastically, had arthritis and no energy, felt awful, and was constipated all the time.

I was really happy to find out about the raw food diet but was hesitant that it would not work due to my hypoglycemia. In the past whenever I tried to go back to being a vegetarian (eating cooked food), my blood sugar would drop drastically. After reading as much as possible, I took a leap of faith and began the raw food lifestyle, going about 60 percent raw. A month after I started I saw you at Loving Life Café in New Oxford, Pennsylvania, and started drinking green smoothies. It has made all the difference in the world! And my husband now drinks them with me whenever I make them. My hypoglycemia is gone; what a relief. I can't tell you the absolute joy I feel every time I eat fruit. My arthritis is gone, I sleep like a baby, my eyesight has improved, and I lost twenty-five pounds; I feel renewed, rejuvenated, and healthy.

In addition to drinking two large green smoothies once or twice a day, I eat raw veggies, fruit, nuts, seeds, and sprouts; avocados and olives for fat along with some nuts, and a big salad for dinner. I have been eating 95 percent raw foods since October of last year. (I eat one cooked meal with my husband every week when we go out for dinner—it seems to make him happy, and I feel like my body can withstand it for one meal.) Thank you for giving the world health and energy.

—*Susan Savia, Pennslyvania*

GET A HOBBY FOR YOUR EXTRA ENERGY

I began my green smoothie adventure in May of 2009. I was introduced to green smoothies by a street vendor named Daniel at our local farmer's market. It was yummy, but more importantly, it was a way for me to get the greens I knew I needed into my life. I was impressed with Daniel's spiel about the healthy benefits of green smoothies, and I took his suggestion to buy *Green for Life*. I was so enthusiastic about what I read that I attended one of Victoria's Joy for Life retreats near Mount Shasta in California. I have since realized that the book is a classic. It has certainly changed my life and the life of my family. We have purchased more than thirty copies of it from RawFamily.com and given them away to friends, doctors, and wellness centers.

After reading *Green for Life* I bought a Vita-Mix blender and began experimenting with my own recipe for green smoothies. Victoria's warning about her invention was right: if you begin drinking green smoothies every day, and I drink about a half gallon daily, you'd better have a hobby to help you burn all the extra energy you will have. I now sleep one hour less every night than before, and I always wake up feeling great. In nine months I have effortlessly lost about twenty-five pounds. I have so much energy that my sixteen year old daughter has had to join a twelve-step group to help her stop rolling her eyes.

I can't believe how it has affected my life. Projects that were unfinished have been easily completed, and I have time to begin doing things I "didn't have time for." My wife and daughter began drinking green smoothies when they witnessed what was happening to me. They are now both hooked as well.

It is my job to purchase the ingredients and to make sure there are always plenty of green smoothies on hand. If I ever fall just a little behind, one of them will comment on how I need to get it in gear and get some made. The girls have become vegetarians, and I am a vegan. I have stopped taking all supplements and vitamins, and of course, due to my vegan diet, I have watched my cholesterol numbers decline dramatically.

Never a day goes by that I don't tell someone about this miracle. I believe that someday, Victoria's secret will become known worldwide as the cure for the health problems caused by the way we eat today.

—*R. J. Jones, San Diego*

DIABETIC CAN EAT FRUIT

It has been nine days since I began eating my dandelion greens and mango smoothie every morning. I want to share the feeling I have inside as I'm eating it. It's almost the same feeling as being thoroughly parched and dehydrated on a hot day, and then how you feel as you drink cold water in abundance. As I eat my green smoothie, I feel like I just cannot get enough—my body wants more and more and more. It is so good and so satisfying.

My blood sugars have been great, although there are no changes with my insulin. I have not eaten fruit since January, so I'm thrilled to have them back and working so well with my diabetes. Thank you both for your passion and for sharing it with me and so many others.

—*Lauren Thompson*

REDUCED CHOLESTEROL

Three months ago my doctor wanted to put me on Lipitor, a hypertension medication, and Fosamax to increase bone density. I am sixty-four years old, so far in good health, and have tried on and off to eat only raw food, but I have not been able to do so for very long. I read about your green smoothie research, bought this book, and was given three months' grace by my MD—who told me a number of times that I would not be able to reduce my cholesterol level of 260 ("no one ever can")—to try green smoothies before the medication. After three months called me and said that my blood test read 223; he appeared to be somewhat stunned. In the short conversation we had, this rather taciturn man used the word *amazing* four times and gave me huge credit three times for my weight loss of twelve pounds and getting my blood pressure down to normal. The smoothies, combined with raw and lightly steamed vegetables, were an easy way to eat even in the last three months of a New York winter.

—*Elisabeth Sheehey, New York*

FROM BEEF AND PORK TO GREEN SMOOTHIE

This testimony goes out to all the big fellows out there. I was the guy who, when given an option of beef or pork in my burrito, said "both, and add some extra cheese while you're at it." I am the guy who was offended at the mention of it costing extra money for extra toppings. The very sight of my obvious excitement at an all-you-can-eat buffet caused the managers to quiver with fear. I was the guy who was shocked when asked if I would like salad with my steak. Salad? Can you imagine? "No, send me some wings instead." I was the one who honestly believed that Rocky Road was not just an ice cream but, for the brave, a way of life. I loved this stuff, and it was killing me.

I was grossly overweight and actually ashamed of myself. That's when my wife started researching about raw foods. One of her friends mentioned green smoothies. I tried one and found it a bit thick but cleverly delicious. Each new dinner creation that my wife presented to me was both refreshing and pleasing to the eye. Don't get me wrong; I wasn't instantly hooked, but after choosing to put my health first, I actually started to like them.

I have been drinking green smoothies for a little more than three weeks now, and I feel more alive than ever. Just the other morning I woke up before my alarm clock! That has happened a few times in a row now. I have never been a morning person, and now I wake up with so much energy. It was almost scary to be so alert, but it was a welcome change. The most exciting thing is that now I crave the good stuff, the greener the better. I have lost a lot of weight. I really don't know how much, but I have gone from a size 48 in pants to a 42 (almost 40) and I'm not done yet. This is all still new for me but I have felt the difference, and I am not going back now that I have the energy and desire to exercise. I know the weight will keep coming off. The food is not only delicious, but for all you super-sizers, it's also surprisingly satisfying. So to you, my friend, I say "jump in." Start living. This is real; this is good; this is right. Some people might say that I am extreme, but I choose to say that I am raw. A big shout-out to Victoria for teaching us how to eat healthy and to drink those delicious green smoothies. More, please!

—*Mr. R. R. V.*

GREEN SMOOTHIE HELPS TO PREPARE
FOR A MARATHON

I've been a raw foodist for over a year and a half now, and over the past few months I have given green smoothies a large role in my diet. I drink at least one almost every day. I'm currently training for my first marathon. Prior to this training, the farthest I had ever run was about three and a half miles. I had not been able to run farther because I always seemed to injure one of my knees, meaning I would have to stop running for weeks until it felt better. I also felt as though I could not possibly push myself to run farther. I'm happy to report that I am now up to fourteen miles (which means I am a half-marathoner!) and not only have I not injured myself, I have not been the least bit sore the day after a run—even after running eight, ten, twelve, or fourteen miles. The other participants in my training group often complain of soreness, and I have been recovering very well. Sometimes I am a bit sore immediately following a run, but I always feel great the next day.

I notice that I have a lot of energy for a workout if I drink a green smoothie as a pre-workout meal. My favorite pre-workout smoothie is banana (or mango) with celery. This provides me with the sugars and electrolytes I need for the long runs in the summer heat.

—*B. E., Chicago*

WHEELCHAIR FOR SALE

Three months ago I considered my life pretty much over. To me, living was a slow dying, and dying was the final end to my suffering. I am twenty-five, and I was in a wheelchair. I couldn't walk the ten feet from my bedroom to the couch in the living room without panting for air and feeling spasms in my back start to take hold. I had been this way for over six months, and I lost every hope of ever being able to walk on my own again. I was beyond miserable; I was more than two hundred pounds overweight. To make matters worse, I also had advanced sleep apnea; it was so bad that I could not even use the CPAP machine that most sufferers use because even at full power it did not provide me enough air to allow me to breathe at night. I never made it to REM sleep at all and most nights frequently woke up two to three times from lack of oxygen. I was beyond conventional help. Because of my poor sleep, I was exhausted all day long, and I would literally fall asleep every five to ten minutes no matter what I was doing or where I was. My life became brief moments of being awake in pain and struggling to function as best I could before I fell asleep again. I was depressed all the time and cried on a daily basis.

Then a month ago my aunt and uncle, who are into raw foods, invited me to come to Oregon and stay with them for a while and try raw foods to see if they could improve my health at all. I figured that I would give it a try—since nothing else had worked, and I was sure that the way I was living and the severity of my health meant I would never see my thirtieth birthday. On my first day, I decided to try to walk, and within less than five minutes I was in tears. My back just wouldn't let me move. That day I went one hundred percent raw and started drinking green smoothies. I pushed myself every day to walk a little further. By the end of the first week I was able to walk the thirty feet to the barn, I could stay awake for hours, and I even felt like I was starting to lose weight. It has been over two weeks now, and I am still one hundred percent raw. I have lost twenty-five pounds, I can stay awake for the whole day, and yesterday I even hiked—yes, hiked—a quarter-mile hill on the farm. I couldn't believe it! When I reached the top I sat down and cried, not because I was in pain, but because I had walked. That is the farthest I have walked in over a year, and it's just the beginning.

My whole attitude has changed, too: I am no longer depressed, and I have a positive outlook now. I feel like a new person inside and out. I know that I have been given a second chance to live and that raw foods saved my life. I will never go back to eating and living the way I was before. Who would want to trade this miracle of life and health for a few moments of indulging bad foods? Definitely not me. I think about all I have accomplished in two short weeks, and I know that in the future I can do anything because I am alive now, I have strength and energy. I would totally urge everyone to give raw foods a chance to help improve the quality of their health and lives. I want everyone to feel as wonderful as I do.

—*J. S., Sacramento*

GREEN SMOOTHIES HELP NORMALIZE B12 LEVEL

I was allergic to all foods to such a degree that I could not sleep. I frequently called emergency services, and in one month I was hospitalized five times. I was diagnosed with chronic fatigue syndrome and hypothyroidism in 1989. I felt confusion and muscle pain for five years, suffered allergies and candida, and was once hospitalized. I couldn't work physically or dance. I wanted to die. I was given high doses of Xanax and antibiotics for a hiatal hernia, which did not help me at all and gave me heart palpitations. At this point I became a vegan, which only made a slight improvement. Then I went on a raw food diet and started to feel a lot better right away. However, my cholesterol was still high at 200. I was 90 percent raw for about seven years. Most of my symptoms were gone except my vitamin B12 level was low. My doctor put me on B12 shots and supplements.

Five months ago I added green smoothies to my diet and my health dramatically improved. I usually drink one quart a day. I like lambsquarters or kale as a base with parsley, pear, mango, and apple. Sometimes I add papaya and soaked chia seeds. After four months my cholesterol dropped to 170, and my thyroid tested normal. The most exciting change was that my B12 level tested normal for the first time in many years, and my doctor said I don't need B12 shots anymore. I love how I feel! The heart murmurs stopped. I have a lot fewer cravings for unhealthy foods. I lost twelve pounds and it feels so good, especially because I am a dancer. I eat two meals a day and have a lot of energy. I vigorously dance swing and polka ten hours a week. My white hair of twenty years is suddenly growing dark again.

At sixty-seven years old I don't fear anything anymore as my life attitude has significantly changed. I've never felt so well balanced in my whole life. My massage therapist told me my skin is glowing and my muscle tone has improved. I look ten years younger, and I feel twenty years younger. Since I incorporated green smoothies into my diet my kids can't keep up with me anymore, and I beat my seventeen-year-old grandson at tennis. At our dance club I outdance a lot of younger dancers. I can do six hours straight of polka, waltzes, or swing. People always ask me what my secret is. Since I carry my green drink everywhere, I am always happy to share.

Many people my age often have severe digestion problems, which I also suffered. Since I began drinking green smoothies my bowels work fantastically; one meal in, one meal out. My kidneys became a lot stronger, and I don't wake up to urinate in the middle of the night anymore. My liver spots have faded noticeably. My eyesight improved so that I don't need my glasses most of the time. I am able to maintain a positive attitude even through the most challenging moments of my life. I feel calmer and more focused. I recently increased my business in Washington, DC, which I run from California, three thousand miles away, using fax, computer, phone, and frequently commute by plane. I also host seven huge potlucks per year with the San Francisco Vegetarian Society and East Bay Vegetarian Society as well as many raw food potlucks and classes. To help other people with healing information I maintain my own Web site, www.LizzysLanding.com.

I am supporting Victoria's research on chimpanzees and everything else she is involved in. I believe that the raw diet with green smoothies added is the future of all nutrition. I admire Victoria's courage and purpose in life to make a healthier planet.

—*Elizabeth Bechtold, California*

HEALING ECZEMA

I am fifty-seven years old, and since childhood I have been very allergic to everything. I was born with eczema and had to take heavy medications all my life. Every night I would scratch my entire body till it was raw and bleeding. I got worse and worse, and the doctors doubled my medication, including steroids. It put out some of the fire but left me bleeding and bruised with ugly rashes all over. I was hospitalized five times for several days, which never helped. Three times I felt so ill that I thought I would die.

The miracle began when my friend Elizabeth introduced me to a so-called green smoothie. This remarkable beverage not only greatly improved my skin condition, but I am also sleeping much better—without scratching myself bloody every night. After only two weeks I truly am feeling more comfortable in my skin, looking better every day. My endless hell is now coming to an end. It is truly a blessing to feel better and to finally become more productive in my life after fifty-seven years of suffering.

—*Karl E. U., California*

REVERSING PANCREATIC CANCER

I am a middle-school teacher of English in Taipei, Taiwan, with a very stressful life. As a result of my annual physical exam, I was told that I had pancreatic cancer, as the CA19-9 test came back at a level of 40; normal is 33. I felt scared, and I didn't want to die. I have two daughters who are still in school and depend entirely on me. Instead of taking a traditional medical route, I tried drinking wheatgrass juice, but I couldn't tolerate the taste at all. I began to eat raw fruits and vegetables and stopped eating meat and dairy products. After three months, I was tested again. The test again came back with a level of 40. Doctors told me that my cancer was not progressing, but it was also not diminishing. Then I read Victoria's book and learned about green smoothies. I began drinking sixteen ounces of the green smoothies daily, and they became a regular part of my daily diet. I usually used orange juice as liquid and added a banana and pineapple or mango. The green was parsley, sunflower sprouts, romaine lettuce, and young pea sprouts. After another three months, when I returned for my follow-up checkup, the CA19-9 test showed a level of 28, better than normal! I believe that green smoothies saved my life.

—*S. Chiao, Taiwan*

INDIGESTION AND CRAVINGS FOR SWEETS ARE GONE

Audrey's and my own experiences are very similar with green smoothies:

1. We have each dropped about five pounds since starting this regimen a couple of months ago. Audrey went from 150 pounds down to 145, and I went from 196 pounds down to 191.

2. We are experiencing great energy along with free and wonderful bowel movements—often three times daily!

3. According to the "acid tests," Audrey, blood type O negative, has plenty of stomach acid naturally and hardly ever experiences indigestion. Hugh, blood type A positive, has very low stomach acid. I took four acid capsules with my regular full meal, and they did the trick with no indigestion from lack of acid and no burning from too much acid. I used to have indigestion every day, depending on baking soda for relief; then I discovered that if I ate a whole orange at the first onset of indigestion, my discomfort would be gone by the time I finished eating it. With the green smoothies I experience no stomach discomfort of any kind. It's wonderful!

4. Our desire for ice cream and sweets has dwindled fast. A nice juicy steak sounds good, and I may salivate a bit thinking of it, but I have no problem in passing it up either. I confess that twice in the past two weeks we were invited to steak barbecues, and twice I went off the wagon—and twice suffered with indigestion afterward. It's just not worth it. After last evening's feast of raw food at our first raw food potluck in Myrtle Creek, Oregon, I ate like a pig after first having a green smoothie before we left home, and I still did not experience any indigestion whatsoever.

—*Hugh and Audrey B.*

GIVEN UP COFFEE

I went through a divorce last year and have been under quite a bit of stress. When I attended my first raw food lecture I had been really stressed out. My digestion had gotten so bad that almost everything I ate caused gas and bloating. My doctor said I was deficient in almost everything because I wasn't absorbing much of anything. So when I was able to participate in the Roseburg Study, I was thrilled. When we first started the study I didn't notice any difference when I got up to the four capsules of HCl with food. I know I have very little stomach acid and have a hard time digesting food. When we started on the smoothies, I often had to use one capsule of HCl just to keep from having what I guessed was heartburn or acid reflux if I was at all stressed. With that, I could digest the smoothie just fine. I didn't notice much the first week, but starting the second week I was amazed. I started waking up before my alarm went off, and that was really something. Usually I could barely wake up and drag myself out of bed even after eight hours of sleep. I was waking up easily and ready to start my day. I hadn't given up all my bad habits like coffee in the morning, cooked foods, and some wine at night, but even doing those "bad" things my energy was much better.

I really started looking forward to the smoothies every day and would have loved to have had more. I just didn't have the time right then to make more of it for myself. Now that school is out and my son's activities have slowed down a bit, I am able to be at home more, so I plan to get myself back into the routine of having green smoothies every day. I know I felt so much better and had more energy.

I have given up coffee now and have turned my coffee grinder into my flax seed grinder. I also noticed that my colon was working better while I was doing the smoothies, so that really helped me feel less toxic as well. Eating raw is something I *know* is the right thing to do; I just have a hard time making it happen. I think that doing the smoothies makes it easier than ever to do the raw thing and to get the nutrients that I am lacking. My digestion is gradually improving, and I did lose two pounds during the month of the study—not a huge weight loss, but a loss nonetheless. I wonder how much I would have lost if I hadn't been doing all the "bad" things at the same time. I needed this push to get back into taking better care of myself, so I thank you for that. Busy moms need better self-care, and doing the green smoothies is how I'm going to do that. I'm looking forward to seeing my health continue to improve and my energy increase. I want to keep up with this teenage boy of mine!

—L. H.

CATARACT REGRESSED FROM FORTY PERCENT TO TEN PERCENT

On October of 2004 I was told that my cholesterol level was so high it was a miracle that I could even get to the doctor's office to hear this terrible news. Parallel to that, arthritis in both my hands was so painful that every morning I was waking up with aches and pains from my crippling hands. I was devastated, since I play the piano and music is a great part of my life. To top it all, my eyesight was getting worse, and a cataract was setting into my left eye. The eye doctor told me that this was a progressive illness and only surgery would help.

What to do? More pills? No. I decided with the help of raw friends to go raw immediately. I went on a trip to Germany, where my family overseas had prepared all kinds of cooked foods and baked cakes for my arrival. I announced to them that on doctor's orders I had to continue raw. A big silence followed, but to my amazement they all respected my wish. I even prepared delicious raw foods there, including desserts. Everyone was astounded and more than pleasantly surprised at the newly discovered taste. I spent four weeks overseas, using the recipes that I had taken with me to keep me going. I had a ball everywhere.

I got back to Toronto and went back for another checkup. The doctor announced to me that my cholesterol was incredibly good compared to that of a young person; I am fifty-eight, so that was another compliment. He said that whatever I was doing was good, so keep on doing it. I share with him my experience with the raw diet, but it went in one ear and out the other.

When I went for my eye examination the doctor was totally taken aback, announcing to me that not only had the cataract regressed from 40 percent to 10 percent, but my eyesight was getting much better. I asked him whether in all his years of practice he had seen a similar case, and his answer was an emphatic no. I told him that I credited this improvement and reversal of sickness to my raw diet. It didn't click with him, but the patients in the waiting room all heard what I shared with my doctor.

I have thrown out all my pills, and I feel so much better now. My energy level is so much higher; I have lost thirty-five pounds and have never looked so good in my life. These are the tangible results after a few months of a raw diet, and I'm wondering about the wonderful rejuvenation my internal organs also must be experiencing.

—*Deanna A. Gontard*

HAPPY DAYS ON RAW FOODS

Before I attended Victoria and Igor's presentation in Riddle, Oregon, I was in a very sad place. I didn't want to be on the planet anymore. I felt so tired, so depressed, so sick. When I heard the enthusiastic presentation by Victoria, my heart smiled. I found new hope, and I found an answer to my problems. I felt inside that eating more fresh fruits and vegetables and greens was right for me and was exactly what I needed. But I didn't know how or if I could do it.

I had so little stomach acid that I was part of the Roseburg Study. Thirty days on green smoothies, and my body wants only raw foods. I feel energy, my vision began to improve, and my joy came back. My blood sugar has stabilized, as have my moods. I want to live! I have energy and regular bowel movements. My vision is clearer, and my skin is healthier. I feel so grateful.

—*Bridget B. W.*

RAW FOOD BABY ZANDER

Arrival of Z: Alexander, alias Zander, alias Z, born in Beaufort, South Carolina, January 1, 2004, six pounds and thirteen ounces, 19.5 inches long. We received the call to come and adopt Zander when he was four days old; the lawyer had been out of town on vacation when Z was born.

First four months: Z's main foods are goat's milk, breast milk from a wet nurse, and water.

Fifth month: we introduced Z to raw food juices.

Sixth month: added barley green juice as well as thinly blended green smoothies in small amounts.

Ninth month: Z loves avocados and apples.

Tenth month: Z prefers to have lemons, apples, and celery in every smoothie.

Eleventh month: Z likes to help me in the kitchen when I make smoothies. He sits on the countertop and hands me things, or I let him stir the contents of the unplugged blender with a large wooden spoon. Z's blood iron level was tested at a high 12.9 percent. Z's doctor said, "Wow! What have you been feeding him, nails?"

Twelfth month: Z began to eat greens-based smoothies. Z likes to try feeding himself and then offers it to us on his spoon. Z still wants milk, and he nearly weaned himself, but he started again when I was gone for a few days.

Fifteenth and sixteenth months: Z's blood iron count remains high. It was last tested at 11.9 percent. Z's pediatrician asked a lot of questions during the last visit. Every answer was resoundingly positive to his ears. The doctor's final words were, "Everything checks out at or above normal. I don't need to recheck him until the twenty-four-month well-patient visit." This means that he recommended skipping the routine eighteen-month checkup.

Since his introduction to green food, Z has had two or three regular bowel movements each day. I'm convinced that the green-based smoothies are keeping his bowels lubricated and hydrated, mostly because of the high water and oil content. The fruit and veggie fiber also stimulates peristalsis. I like the old adage, "Let food be your medicine and medicine be your food."

—*Clare Levin*

LITTLE NICOLAS LIKES IT TOO

I started drinking green smoothies religiously along with my husband, Stephan, when I was about six months pregnant with our son, Nicolas, the first grandson of the Boutenko family. I noticed that I had more energy and had an overall feeling of good health. I also had a wonderful delivery that went smoothly, and the baby did not exhibit the usual signs of distress during contractions, such as a low heartbeat. In fact, every time a contraction started, the baby's heartbeat would not falter in the slightest. After Nicolas was born, I continued the smoothies, and I believe their benefits went directly to him through breastfeeding. He has amazed all of us, including his pediatrician, because he is consistently ahead of the curve in developmental stages and is now trying to walk. Nicolas is almost nine months old, and unlike his peers he has never been sick once. We credit our excellent health to the green smoothie.

—*Tasia, Stephan, and Nicolas Boutenko*

Testimonials of Roseburg Study Participants

To collect more data for my research, I asked the participants of the Roseburg Study to answer the following questions.

1. Was it hard to drink one quart of green smoothie every day?
2. Did the rest of your diet change as a result of the green smoothies?
3. Did you notice any changes in your health?
4. Did your cravings for unhealthy foods lessen?
5. Have you noticed any change in your weight?
6. Did your sleep change?
7. Did your elimination change?
8. Did your energy level change?
9. Did anybody comment on how you looked?
10. Did you have any symptoms of detox?
11. Did you have any negative experiences?
12. Would you like to continue drinking green smoothies?

The answers were so authentic that I decided to include them all in order to reflect the multitude of positive changes that occurred. I took out only the unanswered questions.

Hugh B.

1. Was it hard to drink one quart of green smoothie every day?
   No.

2. Did the rest of your diet change as a result of the green smoothies?
   Yes, I have less desire for other foods.

3. Did you notice any changes in your health?
   Yes; more energy.

4. Did your cravings for unhealthy foods lessen?
   Yes; less ice cream these days.

5. Have you noticed any change in your weight?
   Yes, a slight loss of four pounds.

6. Did your sleep change?
   Yes. Much.

7. Did your elimination change?
   Oh, yes!

8. Did anybody comment on how you looked?
   No. Not to my face, anyway!

9. Did you have any symptoms of detox?
   Not that I can tell—maybe that's why I'm so tired today.

10. Did you have any negative experiences?
    No negatives.

11. Would you like to continue drinking green smoothies?
    Yes. I plan to do so! Great sex.

A. R.

1. Was it hard to drink one quart of green smoothie every day?
   No, I drank more and loved them. My family started drinking them also, and they get upset if I do not make smoothies for them.

2. Did the rest of your diet change as a result of the green smoothies?
   Yes, it made me want to eat raw, and so I am now 95 percent raw. I have not craved junk.

3. Did you notice any changes in your health?
   Yes; I am sleeping well, I have energy, I am positive, I lost ten pounds, and my dandruff healed.

4. Did your cravings for unhealthy foods lessen?
   Yes, I am not craving junk!

5. Have you noticed any change in your weight?
   Yes, I lost ten pounds, but I was also on raw food.

6. Did your sleep change?
   I sleep great! I have had problems with insomnia for years.

7. Did your energy level change?
   I have great energy. I get up at 5 a.m. and feel rested and energetic. I also have an increased sex drive.

8. Did anybody comment on how you looked?
   Yes, my husband and children. I can see a glow on my own face.

9. Did you have any negative experiences?
   Only the mild detox, but I was willing to do it because of the reward.

10. Would you like to continue drinking green smoothies?
    Yes—my whole family is hooked. Thank you so much. I think that green smoothies are one of the most nutritious things we

can ingest. I have been telling my family and friends about it. You have played a part in totally changing my life!

T. T.

1. Was it hard to drink one quart of green smoothie every day?
   No! It was very enjoyable, and I wanted more.

2. Did the rest of your diet change as a result of the green smoothies?
   I wasn't as hungry; I wanted less coffee.

3. Did you notice any changes in your health?
   I had more energy.

4. Did your sleep change?
   Yes, I slept better, longer, and without waking.

5. Did your energy level change?
   I used to have lows around 2 p.m. every day. Now I only have those around once a week or so.

6. Did you have any symptoms of detox?
   I noticed no side effects.

7. Would you like to continue drinking green smoothies?
   I will make my own smoothies and *enjoy* my way to better health. I am thinking about selling green smoothies at my shop.

T. W.

1. Was it hard to drink one quart of green smoothie every day?
   No! I got used to drinking smoothies, and after a week I actually wanted a smoothie.

2. Did the rest of your diet change as a result of the green smoothies?
   Yes. I ate less food at each meal.

3. Did you notice any changes in your health?

Yes. I had more energy and did not take as many afternoon naps. I also did not get hunger pangs before meals and did not get a sugar low in the afternoon.

4. Did your cravings for unhealthy foods lessen?
   A little bit.

5. Have you noticed any change in your weight?
   My weight stayed about the same. I have been working on our five-acre yard, so I already had weight loss.

6. Did your sleep change?
   Yes, right from the first days I slept very soundly and did not grind my teeth at night.

7. Did your elimination change?
   My elimination doubled! Usually it was only once a day, and now it's twice a day very regularly.

8. Did your energy level change?
   Definite increase in energy—I was able to work in the yard and garden all day with just a couple of breaks. Before, I had to take an afternoon nap all the time.

9. Did anybody comment on how you looked?
   We really did not see anyone else, however we did feel much better.

10. Did you have any symptoms of detox?
    Yes, I had stomach cramps on the second round of green smoothies. I was very bloated the first couple of days, but after that, no problem.

11. Did you have any negative experiences?
    No other negative effects.

12. Would you like to continue drinking green smoothies?
    Yes, I will continue drinking green smoothies—I enjoy the flavor and better health, and they are a part of my daily routine.

L. C.

1. Was it hard to drink one quart of green smoothie every day?
   No. I ate it for breakfast, but it was harder at night. Also, I can't eat and drink a lot.

2. Did the rest of your diet change as a result of the green smoothies?
   I'm eating more raw, and I'm trying to find food that is like things I like or crave like bread and cheese.

3. Did your cravings for unhealthy foods lessen?
   No. Some things I wanted badly: textures, flavors, warmth, heat, familiar things. I used to drink coffee, now I do not.

4. Have you noticed any change in your weight?
   I lost four to five pounds.

5. Did your sleep change?
   I sleep more soundly, and I don't get up as often.

6. Did your elimination change?
   It is definitely regular, and I am going more frequently.

7. Did your energy level change?
   I have better energy. I used to get tired at 2 or 3 in the afternoon. I took supplements and drank coffee, but I don't get tired now unless I'm eating more cooked food.

8. Did anybody comment on how you looked?
   Yes, that I looked glowing.

9. Did you have any symptoms of detox?
   Headaches; fever, flu, a bad cold, and bronchitis in the beginning.

10. Did you have any negative experiences?
    Learning to cook raw, I had to use equipment I'm not familiar with. I need food that's fast and easy.

11. Would you like to continue drinking green smoothies?
    Yes. I'm calmer, more peaceful, less anxious.

L. M.

1. Was it hard to drink one quart of green smoothie every day?
   No. I drank more! I made some of my own.

2. Did the rest of your diet change as a result of the green smoothies?
   Yes. I made more smoothies and ate fewer desserts and carbs.

3. Did you notice any changes in your health?
   Yes. I had more energy and lost weight.

4. Did your cravings for unhealthy foods lessen?
   Yes.

5. Have you noticed any change in your weight?
   Yes, I lost nine to eleven pounds.

6. Did your sleep change?
   I sleep a little better.

7. Did your elimination change?
   I urinate more, and I'm less constipated.

8. Did your energy level change?
   I have more energy.

9. Did anybody comment on how you looked?
   Yes.

10. Did you have any symptoms of detox?
    Maybe a mild flu in the beginning.

11. Did you have any negative experiences?
    No.

12. Would you like to continue drinking green smoothies?
    Yes!

Rebeca S.

1. Was it hard to drink one quart of green smoothie every day?
   No, I wish I could have more in a day.

2. Did the rest of your diet change as a result of the green smoothies?
   Yes, I stopped craving sugars and carbohydrates.

3. Did you notice any changes in your health?
   Yes, I feel more energy and no more constipation. It is great!

4. Did your cravings for unhealthy foods lessen?
   Yes.

5. Have you noticed any change in your weight?
   No, definitively no. I am not on one hundred percent raw food yet.

6. Did your sleep change?
   My sleeping is much better.

7. Did your elimination change?
   My bowel movement is great now.

8. Did your energy level change?
   Yes, I have a lot more energy.

9. Did anybody comment on how you looked?
   No, nobody.

10. Did you have any symptoms of detox?
    Only itching: irregular itching all over my body during the first week.

11. Did you have any negative experiences?
    No.

12. Would you like to continue drinking green smoothies?
    Yes, absolutely positively. Thank you very much—I appreciate everything your family has been doing for us.

Brent G.

1. Was it hard to drink one quart of green smoothie every day?
   At first.

2. Did the rest of your diet change as a result of the green smoothies?
   Somewhat; less milk and meat.

3. Did you notice any changes in your health?
   Less fatigue, more energy.

4. Did your cravings for unhealthy foods lessen?
   Yes, except coffee.

5. Have you noticed any change in your weight?
   No.

6. Did your sleep change?
   Yes. I get up earlier and make fewer trips to the bathroom.

7. Did your elimination change?
   My bowel movement improved.

8. Did your energy level change?
   I have the ability to work longer.

9. Did anybody comment on how you looked?
   Yes, they said I looked less stressed.

10. Did you have any symptoms of detox?
    Some: headache and more acne.

11. Did you have any negative experiences?
    No.

12. Would you like to continue drinking green smoothies?
    Yes.

Carrie M.

1. Was it hard to drink one quart of green smoothie every day?
   No, it was easy.

2. Did the rest of your diet change as a result of the green smoothies?
   Yes, I'm eating all raw.

3. Did you notice any changes in your health?
   Yes, I feel disoriented less often when it has been several hours since eating.

4. Did your cravings for unhealthy foods lessen?
   Yes, I had no cravings.

5. Have you noticed any change in your weight?
   Yes. I lost five pounds in the first two weeks, no loss this past week.

6. Did your sleep change?
   It is maybe a little better, but basically the same.

7. Did your elimination change?
   Yes—more frequently, about five times a day.

8. Did your energy level change?
   I have a little more energy, and my mind is a little clearer.

9. Did you have any symptoms of detox?
   Only all the trips to the bathroom. I felt bad one afternoon.

10. Did you have any negative experiences?
    No.

11. Would you like to continue drinking green smoothies?
    I will continue due to a positive blood test on the ANA test.

Mandy O.
(Mom answered for her.)

1. Was it hard to drink one quart of green smoothie every day?
   No.

2. Did you notice any changes in your health?

Yes. She had less asthma—breathing a lot easier than her twin sister, who didn't drink the smoothies (see below).

3. Have you noticed any change in your weight?
   She was 113 pounds, now 110 because it filled her up.

4. Did your energy level change?
   Yes. She has the ability to run longer without being out of breath.

5. Did you have any symptoms of detox?
   No.

Mandy and Becky are seventeen-year-old identical twins. Both are very active and are soccer stars. Mandy drank the green smoothie, and Becky did not. Before starting, Mandy had severe asthma attacks. They were born five weeks premature, and Mandy has had lung problems since birth, which Becky does not.

One week after starting green smoothies, Mandy's asthma attacks stopped. After the second week the girls started running to get a head start for fall soccer. The first time they ran—one mile—during and after the run Becky huffed and puffed like their friends who were running with them. Mandy had very little trouble breathing during and after the run. She felt she was breathing easier and deeper even uphill. They run twice a week after school; Becky huffs and puffs after, but Mandy does not. Becky caught an illness that was going around school, but Mandy did not.

LaVee H.

1. Was it hard to drink one quart of green smoothie every day?
   No. I would have liked more. It was so nice to have the work done for me. Thank you!

2. Did the rest of your diet change as a result of the green smoothies?
   Yes. I was more conscious of eating more raw food each day.

3. Did you notice any changes in your health?

Yes. I had more energy, and I am waking up before my alarm goes off.

4. Did your cravings for unhealthy foods lessen?

Sometimes—stress influenced these cravings more than anything.

5. Have you noticed any change in your weight?

Yes, I lost almost two pounds.

6. Did your sleep change?

Yes. I dream more and wake before my alarm goes off. (I usually sleep OK.)

7. Did your elimination change?

Yes, I'm less constipated—it started more green, then went to more brown.

8. Did your energy level change?

Yes. I have more energy, I woke up more easily in the morning, and I felt happier.

9. Did anybody comment on how you looked?

Yes, one person said I looked good.

10. Did you have any symptoms of detox?

Yes. I had slight nausea or heartburn, which usually happened when I was extremely stressed before drinking the smoothie. I have been going through a lot of emotional things that have been very stressful, so maybe I was detoxing negative emotions more than physical detox.

11. Would you like to continue drinking green smoothies?

Yes. I hope to do even more.

Audrey B.

1. Was it hard to drink one quart of green smoothie every day?

No, it was easy; they are delicious.

2. Did the rest of your diet change as a result of the green smoothies?
   Yes. We cut back a lot and watched what we ate.

3. Did you notice any changes in your health?
   Yes. The green smoothie cleared my system daily.

4. Did your cravings for unhealthy foods lessen?
   Yes. We are working on eliminating ice cream.

5. Have you noticed any change in your weight?
   Yes, a loss—four pounds.

6. Did your sleep change?
   Yes. I slept better and had a deeper sleep.

7. Did your elimination change?
   Yes. You get up, walk, and have to go.

8. Did your energy level change?
   Yes. I'm pleased.

9. Did anybody comment on how you looked?
   Yes. I was told I was glowing. My sex life improved.

10. Did you have any symptoms of detox?
    No symptoms that I felt.

11. Did you have any negative experiences?
    No. None at all.

12. Would you like to continue drinking green smoothies?
    Yes. I definitely plan to do so!

Marion C., age 75

1. Was it hard to drink one quart of green smoothie every day?
   I had no problem drinking one quart daily. I sometimes mixed other fruit juice with it.

2. Did the rest of your diet change as a result of the green smoothies?

With smoothies I take one glass in early in the morning, one about noon, and again in the evening or at bedtime.

3. Did you notice any changes in your health?
   I have noticed no craving for any food. I also notice my fingernails are stronger again.

4. Did your cravings for unhealthy foods lessen?
   Yes. Usually I have had one meal, and smoothies kept me satisfied.

5. Have you noticed any change in your weight?
   No weight change; never has been.

6. Did your sleep change?
   I sleep more soundly now. Before, I could lie for two to three hours before getting to sleep. I used valerian root capsules too.

7. Did your elimination change?
   My bowels have always been very loose and pale yellow in color. Now they are soft, and I may go three times daily. I had no abdominal discomfort.

8. Did your energy level change?
   I used to need a rest in the afternoon. Now I can keep busy all day with occasional breaks, so it seems like I have more energy for activities like caring for the goats and llamas, gardening, and spreading crushed rock and wood chips for landscaping. I definitely have more energy.

9. Did you have any symptoms of detox?
   No. No bad reaction whatsoever.

10. Did you have any negative experiences?
    No.

11. Would you like to continue drinking green smoothies?
    I have had some heart arrhythmia for several years and am taking multifood supplements. I have been taking Mannatech food supplements since December 2004 and have noticed my heart

rhythm return to normal. I also have had cold hands and feet and minimal energy, but all these minor problems have disappeared. I have always thought that I may have a hypothyroid condition, but something I'm doing is good, so I am happy and plan to remain on smoothies.

Gabrielle R., age 35

1. Was it hard to drink one quart of green smoothie every day?
   Yes, I did have to break it into small portions. The taste was fine, but I did have trouble with the thickness and quantity as well as too little variety, but I will experiment on my own.

2. Did the rest of your diet change as a result of the green smoothies?
   Yes, I ate less in general. I craved less junk food and more fruits and raw foods.

3. Did you notice any changes in your health?
   Yes, I have more energy! I require less sleep, my temperament is more even and pleasant, I had none of my usual PMS symptoms, and my skin cleared up beautifully.

4. Did your cravings for unhealthy foods lessen?
   Yes. I was able to drop many unhealthy items from my diet fairly easily.

5. Have you noticed any change in your weight?
   I only lost less than five pounds by the scale, but I do feel as thought I lost a bit more.

6. Did your sleep change?
   I sleep better and require less sleep per night. I wake up fully awake and don't linger in bed as I used to.

7. Did your elimination change?
   I definitely go more than ever before, and I definitely am urinating more frequently. I didn't notice any specific color changes.

8. Did your energy level change?

Yes. I find each evening that everything I set out to do each day actually got done! I don't have work piled up undone at the end of the day as I would before.

9. Did anybody comment on how you looked?

I did have just a couple of mild compliments.

10. Did you have any symptoms of detox?

I did have mild mucus coughing and through the sinuses, as well as mild nausea the first few days.

11. Did you have any negative experiences?

No!

12. Would you like to continue drinking green smoothies?

Definitely. I look forward to experimenting with various recipes and sharing them with my family.

Leah W.

1. Was it hard to drink one quart of green smoothie every day?

No, however I wouldn't want more.

2. Did the rest of your diet change as a result of the green smoothies?

I did eat more veggies as I was more aware of "good" foods.

3. Did you notice any changes in your health?

No constipation at all, fresher taste in foods, possibly more energy.

4. Did your cravings for unhealthy foods lessen?

It filled me up so that I ate less other food, but I could still desire other foods.

5. Did your elimination change?

I usually have one BM per day, but with smoothies I had two or more with no constipation.

6. Did your energy level change?
   Before smoothies I would eat dinner and then sit and watch TV and fall asleep. After smoothies I didn't fall asleep watching TV.

7. Would you like to continue drinking green smoothies?
   Yes! I will try to continue and experiment with different greens, adding more organic produce as well. Thank you so much for exposing me to raw foods, greens, and better nutrition!

Al C.

1. Was it hard to drink one quart of green smoothie every day?
   No. I could do more easily.

2. Did the rest of your diet change as a result of the green smoothies?
   Yes. I've started to eat a lot more salads, but occasionally I still get cravings.

3. Did you notice any changes in your health?
   I've lost about five to six pounds.

4. Did your cravings for unhealthy foods lessen?
   I seem to eat far less junk.

5. Have you noticed any change in your weight?
   I've lost about five to six pounds.

6. Did your sleep change?
   I seem to toss and turn less, as my hair isn't as messy in the morning when I wake up.

7. Did your elimination change?
   I went three to four times daily. It felt like my whole colon was emptying all at once.

8. Did your energy level change?
   Not a really noticeable change yet; it seems about the same.

9. Did you have any negative experiences?
   No.

10. Would you like to continue drinking green smoothies?
    I will continue, yes. I am fifty-four, and I definitely noticed a significant improvement in my male response—about fifteen years' worth.

Wib

1. Did the rest of your diet change as a result of the green smoothies?
   Yes, I ate less prepared food.

2. Did you notice any changes in your health?
   Yes, three pounds of weight loss.

3. Did your cravings for unhealthy foods lessen?
   Yes. They were maybe motivational rather than from taste.

4. Did your sleep change?
   Yes, I rested more consistently.

5. Did your elimination change?
   Bowel movements were more regular, and urine was more sensational.

6. Did you have any symptoms of detox?
   Mild headaches.

7. Did you have any negative experiences?
   I never did enjoy the taste; I just drank it for the test and health's sake.

8. Would you like to continue drinking green smoothies?
   Yes, in various degrees and kinds of drinks and preparations. We will not be going one hundred percent raw; hopefully 75 to 90 percent raw. But thanks for your focus and help.

Dee S.

1. Was it hard to drink one quart of green smoothie every day?
   No.

2. Did the rest of your diet change as a result of the green smoothies?
   Yes, I ate mostly raw.

3. Did your cravings for unhealthy foods lessen?
   Yes.

4. Have you noticed any change in your weight?
   Yes, I lost ten pounds.

5. Did anybody comment on how you looked?
   A few people noticed weight loss.

6. Did you have any symptoms of detox?
   Not that I was aware of.

7. Did you have any negative experiences?
   Nothing negative.

Terri B., age 51

1. Was it hard to drink one quart of green smoothie every day?
   No, it was easy and enjoyable. More would have been nice.

2. Did the rest of your diet change as a result of the green smoothies?
   Yes, my family and I have started eating some raw.

3. Did you notice any changes in your health?
   Yes, I have more energy, and my husband is easier to get along with.

4. Did your cravings for unhealthy foods lessen?
   Yes, my cravings are almost gone. When I had a lot of bad choices available, I didn't care and did not eat.

5. Have you noticed any change in your weight?
   Yes, I have lost eighteen to twenty pounds.

6. Did your sleep change?
   I was rested, but I did get up more often to use the restroom to urinate.

7. Did your elimination change?
   Yes, I eliminated a lot more than I consumed, and it was easy and gentle.

8. Did your energy level change?
   Yes, I no longer desire a nap whenever time is available.

9. Did you have any symptoms of detox?
   Yes. I had burning eyes and lips as well as headaches.

10. Did you have any negative experiences?
    No—it has been very positive. We are starting to go raw, and trying to figure out how to prepare food for six people (four of them growing boys) is a bit overwhelming.

11. Would you like to continue drinking green smoothies?
    Yes.

Berta D.

1. Was it hard to drink one quart of green smoothie every day?
   No.

2. Did the rest of your diet change as a result of the green smoothies?
   No. I think I crave sugar a little less.

3. Did you notice any changes in your health?
   No. My weight is yo-yoing.

4. Did your energy level change?
   I'm walking a little more, and I've joined Curves.

5. Did anybody comment on how you looked?
   No one commented.

6. Did you have any symptoms of detox?
   No.

7. Did you have any negative experiences?
   No negative experiences.

8. Would you like to continue drinking green smoothies?
   I have more positive than negative in all this experience.

Sunny D.

1. Was it hard to drink one quart of green smoothie every day?
   No, not at all—I could drink them all day long.

2. Did you notice any changes in your health?
   I noticed an improvement in my skin, especially on days when I did not eat other junk.

3. Did your cravings for unhealthy foods lessen?
   A little bit; I had less interest in chocolate.

4. Have you noticed any change in your weight?
   No, it stayed the same.

5. Did your sleep change?
   I sleep better, especially if I don't eat spicy food in addition to smoothies.

6. Did your elimination change?
   There was a slight increase in volume.

7. Did your energy level change?
   I didn't notice a change in energy.

8. Did you have any symptoms of detox?
   I had detox headaches for a night and a day.

9. Did you have any negative experiences?
   None!

10. Would you like to continue drinking green smoothies?
    Definitely! I had already been drinking a huge smoothie daily: forty-eight ounces, approximately 75 to 80 percent fruit with some greens, which I continued to drink for this whole month in addition to the green smoothies. Now I will definitely be continuing the higher-greens type smoothies—I would miss the greens too much if I stopped!

Cindy S.

1. Was it hard to drink one quart of green smoothie every day?
   No—sometimes I wanted more.

2. Did the rest of your diet change as a result of the green smoothies?
   I wanted more fresh food—cooked food wasn't as appealing.

3. Did you notice any changes in your health?
   I was hungrier at meal times the first week or two. I had more regular bowel movements.

4. Did your cravings for unhealthy foods lessen?
   Yes. I wasn't as hungry for sweets, and I was more motivated to eat healthier.

5. Have you noticed any change in your weight?
   I have lost some weight—I like it!

6. Did your sleep change?
   I may be getting by with less sleep.

7. Did your elimination change?
   I had more regular bowel movements: larger in size, and toward the end I noticed darker stools, perhaps getting rid of older accumulation?

8. Did your energy level change?
   I felt good knowing I was doing something so good for myself.

My life is very busy and hectic, and I'm sure if I were more disciplined, I would benefit more.

9. Did anybody comment on how you looked?
No one said anything, except my husband says I play the piano better now!

10. Did you have any symptoms of detox?
None that I know of.

11. Did you have any negative experiences?
None. I enjoyed very much being a part of this study and telling others about it.

12. Would you like to continue drinking green smoothies?
Yes. I want to keep this up.

Vickie G. of Glide, Oregon

1. Was it hard to drink one quart of green smoothie every day?
At first it was, then I got used to the taste. It got easier, and drinking more, I wanted more.

2. Did the rest of your diet change as a result of the green smoothies?
Some; I was occasionally hungrier.

3. Did you notice any changes in your health?
Yes.

4. Did your cravings for unhealthy foods lessen?
Yes. I desire less chocolate and sweets at work.

5. Did your sleep change?
I'm sleeping deeper and dreaming for the first time in almost a year.

6. Did your elimination change?
It is more frequent. I used to have hard pebbles every time I went. Now it is larger, softer, and still more frequent. I'm very thirsty now.

7. Did your energy level change?

   Yes. I take fewer and shorter naps. I work 6 p.m. to 6 a.m., and I am more awake and alert at work; I also have more energy at work.

8. Did anybody comment on how you looked?

   I did—I saw fewer dark wrinkles under my eyes and less puffiness.

9. Did you have any symptoms of detox?

   Yes. I had some headaches in the first weeks, but now I feel better. At first, my acid reflux went away, then I had severe acid even in my mouth, and now I have no acid reflux.

10. Did you have any negative experiences?
    No.

11. Would you like to continue drinking green smoothies?

    Yes, I have a desire to start my own harvesting and doing it on my own. At work, colds and flu go around and around, and I usually got sick too. I haven't gotten sick since starting. Also, my five-year-old drinks it too and likes it.

Bridget H.

1. Was it hard to drink one quart of green smoothie every day?

   It was very easy to drink. It's not hard at all to drink green smoothies.

2. Did the rest of your diet change as a result of the green smoothies?

   My body wanted raw foods starting around the ninth day of drinking green smoothies. I want to be on one hundred percent raw foods soon.

3. Did you notice any changes in your health?

   I had increased energy, motivation to exercise more, my joy came back, my depression lifted, and I don't have suicidal thoughts, along with less blood sugar fluctuation.

4. Did your cravings for unhealthy foods lessen?
   My cravings are almost gone for alcohol, sweets, and chocolate. Thank goodness!

5. Have you noticed any change in your weight?
   I lost a few pounds that I had wanted to lose.

6. Did your sleep change?
   A few times I needed less sleep, and I get up less in the night.

7. Did your elimination change?
   I have been going to the bathroom more times each day. For one and a half weeks I have had very loose bowels, and some diarrhea in the mornings.

8. Did your energy level change?
   I have more energy. I wake up and jog at 6 a.m. before work at 7 a.m.

9. Did anybody comment on how you looked?
   Someone thought I had lost weight and looked fine. I inspired some others with my enthusiasm.

10. Did you have any symptoms of detox?
    I had spots like pimples or a rash (not hives). I had flu symptoms, some nausea when I would think about taking vitamins, diarrhea almost every morning for ten days or so, and a few aches and pains in my joints.

11. Did you have any negative experiences?
    Nothing negative at all.

12. Would you like to continue drinking green smoothies?
    Yes! And I want to be one hundred percent raw too.

Green Smoothie Recipes

IMPORTANT TIPS

Storage of Green Smoothies

While fresh is always best, green smoothies will keep in cool temperatures for up to three days, which can be handy at work and while traveling.

Rotation of Greens

I would like to emphasize the importance of using a wide variety of greens. Try out as many different greens as you can. If you continue to use the same greens, you can expect to lose your desire for green smoothies. It's also important to rotate your greens to avoid a buildup of alkaloids from the same plant—as mentioned earlier, they are perfectly healthy in small quantities but we should moderate our intake. For so many reasons, variety is the spice of life!

Sweet Green Smoothies

❧ WELCOME SMOOTHIE FOR BEGINNERS

Blend well:

1 cup chard
1 cup spinach
8–10 strawberries, stems included
1 mango, peeled
1 apple
1 banana
Juice of 1 lemon
2 cups water

YIELDS 2 QUARTS

❧ HAWAIIAN DANDELION

Blend well:

3 cups dandelion greens
1 cup sweet Hawaiian pineapple
1 banana
1 apple
2 cups water

YIELDS 2 QUARTS

❧ BANAN-DELION

Blend well:

3 cups dandelion greens
4 bananas
1 lime, with peel
3 cups water

YIELDS 2 QUARTS

❧ MINTI-DANDELION

Blend well:

3 cups dandelion greens
1 pint strawberries
2 ripe bananas
1 sprig mint
2 cups water

YIELDS 2 QUARTS

❧ ALOE-HA

Blend well:

1 leaf aloe vera, with peel
2 stalks celery
2 cups kale
1 apple
2 bananas
1 lime, with peel
2 cups water

YIELDS 2 QUARTS

❧ WILD MORNING SMOOTHIE

Blend well:

1 cup mallow (also known as *Malva*)
1 cup sorrel
1 cup stinging nettles
2 pears
2 bananas
2 cups water

YIELDS 2 QUARTS

❧ MERRY GRASSHOPPER

Blend well:

1 cup wheat grass
2 bananas
1 lemon, juiced
½ inch ginger
2 cups water

YIELDS 1 QUART

❧ SWEET FENNEL

Blend well:

1 cup fennel greens
1 cup dandelion greens
1 cup chard
1 pear
1 mango, peeled
1 banana
2 cups water

YIELDS 2 QUARTS

❧ RAW FAMILY WILD BANANGO

Blend well:

2 cups lambsquarters (or plantain,
   chickweed, or other weed)
1 banana
1 mango
2 cups water

YIELDS 1 QUART

✖ VALYA'S FAVORITE

Blend well:

8 leaves romaine lettuce

5 cups watermelon

1 cup water

YIELDS 1 QUART

✖ GREEN BENEVOLENCE

Blend well:

6–8 leaves romaine lettuce

1 cup red grapes

1 medium orange

1 banana

2 cups water

YIELDS 1 QUART

✖ SWEET AND SOUR

Blend well:

6–8 leaves red leaf lettuce

4 apricots

1 banana

¼ cup blueberries

2 cups water

YIELDS 1 QUART

❧ FRESHNESS

Blend well:

6–8 leaves romaine lettuce
½ medium-sized honeydew
2 cups water

YIELDS 1 QUART

❧ ALOE LIVE

Blend well:

1 cup apple juice
1 banana
1 mango
1 small piece aloe
5 leaves kale
2 cups water

YIELDS 1 QUART

❧ SUMMER DELIGHT

Blend well:

6 peaches
2 handfuls spinach leaves
2 cups water

YIELDS 1 QUART

❧ WEEDS FOR KIDS

Blend well:

4 mangoes, peeled
1 handful lambsquarters (or stinging nettles,
    purslane, or other weed)

2 cups water

YIELDS 1 QUART OF SWEET THICK SMOOTHIE, LIKE
PUDDING

❧ STRAWBERRY FIELD

Blend well:

1 cup strawberries
2 bananas
½ bunch romaine lettuce
2 cups water

YIELDS 1 QUART

❧ KIWI ENJOYMENT

Blend well:

4 very ripe kiwis, green or golden
1 ripe banana
3 stalks celery
2 cups water

YIELDS 1 QUART

❧ IGOR'S FAVORITE

Blend well:

½ bunch spinach
4 apples, peeled
½ lime with peel
1 banana
2 cups water

YIELDS 1 QUART

❧ MINTY THRILL

Blend well:

4 ripe pears
4–5 leaves kale
½ bunch mint
2 cups water

YIELDS 1 QUART

❧ TEN FINGERS

Blend well:

10 finger bananas
2 handfuls spinach leaves
2 cups water

YIELDS 1 QUART

❧ RASPBERRY DREAM

Blend well:

2 Bosc pears
1 handful raspberries
4–5 leaves kale
2 cups water

YIELDS 1 QUART

Savory Green Smoothies

❧ SPICY STINGING NETTLES SOUP

Blend well:

1 cup stinging nettles
2 stalks celery

1 cup fresh parsley
1 cup garlic greens
Juice of 1 lemon
1 red bell pepper
1 medium-sized tomato
1 avocado
2 cups water

YIELDS 2 QUARTS

❧ CREAMY GINGER SPINACH

Blend well:

2 cups spinach
1 Bosc pear
1 apple
½ avocado
1 inch ginger
2 cups water

YIELDS 1½ QUARTS

❧ CILANTRO SPICY SOUP

Blend well:

2 cups cilantro
2 stalks celery
5–7 leaves romaine lettuce
4 tomatoes
1 avocado
Juice of 1 lemon
½ jalapeño pepper
2 cups water

YIELDS 2 QUARTS

✜ DILL-OREGANO SOUP

Blend well:

1 cup dandelion greens

5–7 leaves romaine lettuce

1 cucumber

1 avocado

1 cup garlic greens

½ cup dill weed

½ cup oregano

Juice of 2 limes

3 cups water

YIELDS 2 QUARTS

✜ MEDITERRANEAN GREEN

Blend well:

2 cups arugula

3 stalks celery, with leaves

4–5 medium-size ripe tomatoes

1 avocado

½ cup basil

Juice of 1 lemon

½ jalapeño pepper

2 cups water

YIELDS 2 QUARTS

MUSTARD-CILANTRO SOUP

Blend well:

2 cups mustard greens

1 cup cilantro

2 medium-sized ripe tomatoes
Juice of 1 lemon
1 avocado
2 cups water

YIELDS 2 QUARTS

❧ SUPER CILANTRO

Blend well:

4 cups cilantro
1 red bell pepper
1 cup cherry tomatoes
1 avocado
Juice of 1 lemon
1 pear
2 cups water

YIELDS 2 QUARTS

❧ VICTORIA'S FAVORITE

Blend well:

6 leaves red leaf lettuce
¼ bunch fresh basil
Juice of ½ lime
½ red onion
2 stalks celery
¼ avocado
2 cups water

YIELDS 1 QUART

ᴔ SERGEI'S FAVORITE

Blend well:

5 leaves green kale
½ bunch fresh dill
Juice of ½ lime
3 cloves garlic
¼ cup sun-dried tomatoes
2 cups water

YIELDS 1 QUART

ᴔ ORION'S LEMON JALAPEÑO FRESCA

Blend well:

Juice of ½ lemon
4 Roma tomatoes
²/₃ bunch kale
½ inch jalapeño pepper
1 small clove garlic
2 cups water

YIELDS 1 QUART

ᴔ SHAKTI'S GREEN THAI

Blend well:

2½ cups spinach
½ bunch cilantro
1 clove garlic
½ red bell pepper
Juice of ½ lime
1 teaspoon stevia (1 green leaf)
3 Roma tomatoes

2 cups water

<small>YIELDS 1 QUART</small>

⅌ GREEN DELICIOUS

The whole point in making green smoothies is to consume more greens, especially without salt. We include salt in this extraordinarily tasty recipe, however. We found it useful for treating those of our friends who eat a mainstream diet.

Blend well:

5 leaves purple kale

¼ avocado

3 cloves garlic

Juice of ½ lime

2 cups water

½ teaspoon salt

2 Roma tomatoes

<small>YIELDS 1 QUART</small>

⅌ NUTRITIOUSLY BITTER

Blend well:

5 leaves green or purple kale

¼ avocado

3 cloves garlic

¼ cup lime juice

1 bell pepper

2 stalks celery

½ bunch Italian parsley

2 cups water

<small>YIELDS 1 QUART</small>

Super Green Smoothie

❧ VICTORIA'S DREAM

Blend well:

4 cups dandelion greens
2 medium-sized ripe tomatoes
2 cups water

YIELDS 1½ QUARTS

Puddings

❧ BEGINNERS FAVORITE PUDDING

Blend well:

1 cup chard
1 apple
1 banana
1 sprig mint
4–5 dates
2 teaspoons psyllium husk powder
2 cups water

YIELDS 2 QUARTS

❧ CELERY-PAPAYA PUDDING

Blend well:

5 stalks celery
1 Hawaiian papaya, peeled and seeded
1 cup crimson grapes
½ cup spinach

Garnish with sliced fruit.

YIELDS 1 QUART

❧ GREEN VANILLA PUDDING

A children's favorite.

Blend well:

1 cup chard
1 banana
1 apple
1 fresh vanilla bean
1 small Meyer lemon, with peel

Serve in nice glasses; decorate with fresh fruit.

YIELDS 1 QUART

❧ PERSIMMON CINNAMON PUDDING

Blend well:

5–6 ripe persimmons, any variety
2 cups chard
1 banana
2–3 tablespoons water
½ teaspoon cinnamon
½ teaspoon nutmeg

YIELDS 1 QUART

❧ BLUEBERRY PUDDING

Blend well:

1 stalk celery
2 cups fresh blueberries
1 banana
2 cups water

YIELDS 1 QUART

TWO-LAYER PUDDING

A children's favorite.

BOTTOM LAYER

2 cups kale

2 ripe bananas

1 lime, with peel

¼ cup raisins

2 teaspoons psyllium husk powder

2 cups water

*Blend well and quickly pour into 8–10 cups;
fill only halfway.*

TOP LAYER

2 cups kale

2 ripe bananas

2 limes, with peel

¼ cup raisins

1 cup blackberries

2 teaspoons psyllium husk powder

2 cups water

*Blend well and quickly pour onto the bottom
layer. Decorate with fresh fruit or berries.*

YIELDS 8–10 ATTRACTIVE AND DELICIOUS CUPS

SPINACH KUMQUAT PARADISE PUDDING

Excellent for beginners and children.

Blend well:

2 cups baby spinach

6–7 kumquats, with peel and seeds

1 pear
2 bananas
½ cup water

You will likely need to use your tamper to help this mixture blend. Decorate with fresh fruit.

YIELDS 5 CUPS

❧ MANGO-PARSLEY PUDDING

Blend well:

2 large mangoes, peeled
1 bunch parsley
2 cups water

YIELDS 1 QUART

❧ CHIA SEED GREEN PUDDING

Blend well:

1 cup chia jell (1 tablespoon chia seeds
   soaked for 1 hour in 1 cup water)
4 apples, a sweet and juicy variety,
   peeled
Juice of ½ lemon
4–5 leaves kale
1 sprig mint (optional)
2 cups water

YIELDS 1½ QUARTS

NOTES

CHAPTER 3

1. Chimpanzee and Human Communication Institute, 2004, www.cwu.
edu/~cwuchci/faq.html.

2. Derek E. Wildman et al., "Implications of Natural Selection in Shaping
99.4% Nonsynonymous DNA Identity Between Humans and Chimpanzees:
Enlarging Genus *Homo*," *Proceedings of the National Academy of Sciences* 100
(May 19, 2003): 2172.

3. Ibid.

4. James Q. Jacobs, "A Comparison of Some Similar Chimpanzee and
Human Behaviors," *Paleoanthropology in the 1990s* (2000), www.jqjacobs.net.

5. World Wildlife Fund, "Chimpanzees," 2005, http://intothewild.tripod.
com/chimpanzees.htm.

6. Louis R. Sibal and Kurt J. Samson, "Nonhuman Primates: A Critical Role
in Current Disease Research," *ILAR Journal* 42(2), 2001, http://dels.nas.edu/
ilar/jour_online/42_2/nhprole.asp.

7. Ibid.

8. Chimpanzee and Human Communication Institute, 2004, www.cwu.
edu/~cwuchci/faq.html.

9. Nancy Lou Conklin-Brittain, Richard W. Wrangham, and Catherine
C. Smith, "Relating Chimpanzee Diets to Potential Australopithecus Diets,"
Department of Anthropology, Harvard University, 1998, www.cast.uark.edu/
local/icaes/conferences/wburg/posters/nconklin/conklin.html.

10. Jane Goodall, *The Chimpanzees of Gombe,* (Cambridge, MA: Belknap, 1986).

CHAPTER 4

1. Weston A. Price, *Nutrition and Physical Degeneration* 6th ed. (Lemon Grove, CA: Price-Pottenger Nutrition Foundation, 2003).

2. Ibid.

CHAPTER 5

1. U.S. Department of Agriculture Agricultural Research Service, "USDA National Nutrient Database for Standard Reference, Release 18," 2005, www.nal. usda.gov.

CHAPTER 6

1. Herbert M. Shelton, *Dr. Shelton's Hygienic Review* (Pomeroy, WA: Health Research, 1996).

2. Dietary Reference Intakes for males aged 19–30. National Research Council, "Protein and Amino Acids," *Recommended Dietary Allowances* 10th ed. (USDA SR17, 1989).

CHAPTER 7

1. Nancy Lou Conklin-Brittain, Richard W. Wrangham, and Catherine C. Smith, "Relating Chimpanzee Diets to Potential Australopithecus Diets," Department of Anthropology, Harvard University, 1998, www.cast.uark.edu/ local/icaes/conferences/wburg/posters/nconklin/conklin.html.

2. Data for the average adult male aged 19–31 and weighing 170 pounds. National Research Council, "Protein and Amino Acids," *Recommended Dietary Allowances* 10th ed. (USDA SR17, 1989).

3. Joel Fuhrman, *Eat to Live: The Revolutionary Formula for Fast and Sustained Weight Loss* (New York: Little Brown, 2003), 138.

4. W. A. Walker and K. J. Isselbacher, "Uptake and Transport of Macro-molecules by the Intestine: Possible Role in Clinical Disorders," *Gastroenterology* 67 (1974): 531–550.

5. Julia Ross, *The Diet Cure* (New York: Penguin, 1999).

6. U.S. Department of Agriculture Agricultural Research Service, "USDA National Nutrient Database for Standard Reference, Release 18," 2005, www.nal. usda.gov.

7. T. Colin Campbell, *The China Study* (Dallas: BenBella, 2004).

CHAPTER 8

1. Bernard Jensen, *Tissue Cleansing through Bowel Management* (Escondido, CA: Bernard Jensen, 1981).

2. Deepak Chopra, *Perfect Health: The Complete Mind Body Guide* (New York: Three Rivers, 2000).

3. Nancy Lou Conklin-Brittain, Richard W. Wrangham, and Catherine C. Smith, "Relating Chimpanzee Diets to Potential Australopithecus Diets," Department of Anthropology, Harvard University, 1998, www.cast.uark.edu/local/icaes/conferences/wburg/posters/nconklin/conklin.html.

4. Albert Mosséri, *Le jeûne: meilleur remède de la nature* (Geneva: Aquarius, 1993).

5. American Heart Association, "Fiber," www.americanheart.org.

6. Alan M. Tooshi, *Dr. Tooshi's High Fiber Diet* (Lincoln, NE: iUniverse.com, 2001).

7. Myron Winick, *The Fiber Prescription* (New York: Ballantine, 1992).

8. American Heart Association, 2004, www.americanheart.org.

CHAPTER 9

1. Bernard Jensen, *The Healing Power of Chlorophyll* (Escondido, CA: Bernard Jensen, 1981).

2. Walter B. Cannon, *The Wisdom of the Body* (New York: Peter Smith, 1932).

CHAPTER 10

1. W. A. Walker and K. J. Isselbacher, "Uptake and Transport of Macro-molecules by the Intestine: Possible Role in Clinical Disorders," *Gastroenterology* 67 (1974): 531–550.

2. Anil Minocha and David Carroll, *Natural Stomach Care: Treating and Preventing Digestive Disorders with the Best of Eastern and Western Healing Therapies* (New York: Penguin, 2003).

3. Elson M. Haas, *Staying Healthy With Nutrition* (Berkeley, CA: Celestial Arts, 1992).

4. Nancy Lou Conklin-Brittain, Richard W. Wrangham, and Catherine C. Smith, "Relating Chimpanzee Diets to Potential Australopithecus Diets," Department of Anthropology, Harvard University, 1998, www.cast.uark.edu/local/icaes/conferences/wburg/posters/nconklin/conklin.html.

5. www.newswithviews.com/Howenstine/james21.htm.

6. Stephen Stiteler, *A Closer Look at Hypochlorhydria* (Tustin, CA: Institute of Bio-terrain Sciences, 2003).

7. Theodore A. Baroody Jr., *Alkalize or Die* (Portland, OR: Eclectic, 1991).

8. Ibid.

CHAPTER 12

1. "Cancer Now the Top Killer of Americans," *USA Today,* January 20, 2005.

2. Otto Warburg, *The Prime Cause and Prevention of Cancer* 2nd. ed. (Würtzburg, Germany: Konrad Triltsch, 1969), trans. Dean Burk, National

Cancer Institute, Bethesda, MD, http://healingtools.tripod.com/primecause2. html. Lecture delivered to Nobel Laureates on June 30, 1966, at Lindau, Germany.

3. Ibid.

4. Theodore A. Baroody Jr., *Alkalize or Die* (Portland, OR: Eclectic, 1991).

CHAPTER 13

1. Peter Tompkins and Christopher Bird, *The Secret Life of Plants* (New York: Harper and Row, 1989).

2. Peter Tompkins and Christopher Bird, *Secrets of the Soil* (Anchorage: Earthpulse, 2002).

3. Peter Tompkins and Christopher Bird, *The Secret Life of Plants* (New York: Harper and Row, 1989).

4. Organic farm inspector Vyapaka Dasa, *It Ain't Just Dirt!,* 2005, www.hkrl. com/soils.html.

5. C. Benbrook, X. Zhao, J. Yanez, N. Davies, and P. Andrews, "New Evidence Confirms the Nutritional Superiority of Plant-Based Organic Foods," The Organic Center, Boulder, 2008.

6. Peter Tompkins and Christopher Bird, *Secrets of the Soil* (Anchorage: Earthpulse, 2002).

7. David Blume, "Food and Permaculture," www.permaculture.com/node/141.

8. Ibid.

9. Louis Kervran, *Biological Transmutations* (London: Crosby Lockwood, 1972).

10. Peter Tompkins and Christopher Bird, *The Secret Life of Plants* (New York: Harper and Row, 1989).

11. Ibid.

12. P. A. Korolkov, *Spontaneous Metamorphism of Minerals and Rocks* (Moscow: Nauka, 1972).

CHAPTER 14

1. Otto Warburg, "The Oxygen-transferring Ferment of Respiration," 1931 Nobel Prize lecture, *Nobel Lectures, Physiology or Medicine 1922–1941* (Amsterdam: Elsevier, 1965).

2. Patricia Egner, Jin-Bing Wang, et al., "Chlorophyllin Reduces Aflatoxin Indicators among People at High Risk for Liver Cancer," *Proceedings of the National Academy of Sciences* 98 (November 27, 2001).

3. S. Chernomorsky et al., "Effect of Dietary Chlorophyll Derivatives on Mutagenesis and Tumor Cell Growth," *Teratogenesis, Carcinogenesis, and Mutagenesis* 79 (1999): 313–322.

4. M. Vlad et al., *Effect of Cuprofilin on Experimental Atherosclerosis,* Institute of Public Health and Medical Research, University of Medicine and Pharmacy, Cluj-Napoca, Romania, 1995.

CHAPTER 15

1. Vladimir Soloukhin, *Razryv-trava* (Moscow: Molodaya Gvardiya, 2001).

2. Jane Goodall, *The Chimpanzees of Gombe* (Cambridge, MA: Belknap, 1986).

3. Elizabeth Baker, *Unbelievably Easy Sprouting!* (Poulsbo, WA: privately printed, 2000).

CHAPTER 16

1. J. P. Infante R. C. Kirwan, and J. T. Brenna, "High levels of docosahexaenoic acid (22:6*n*-3)-containing phospholipids in high-frequency contraction muscles of hummingbirds and rattlesnakes," *Comparative Biochemistry and Physiology Part B: Biochemistry and Molecular Biology* 130, no. 3 (October 2001)

2. W. E. Lands, "Please don't tell me to die faster," *Inform* 13 (2002):896–897

3. Susan Allport, *The Queen of Fats: Why Omega-3s Were Removed from the Western Diet and What We Can Do to Replace Them* (Berkeley: University of California Press, 2006).

4. "The Agriculture Fact Book 2001–2002," *United States Department of Agriculture.*

5. J. B. Allred, "Too much of a good thing? An overemphasis on eating low-fat foods may be contributing to the alarming increase," *J Am Diet Assoc.* (1995).

6. www.mindfully.org/Water/Fish-Farming-Overtake-Cattle.htm

7. http://earthobservatory.nasa.gov/Features/Phytoplankton/

8. http://nutritiondata.self.com/facts/finfish-and-shellfish-products/4256/2

9. Artemis P. Simopoulos., *The Omega Diet: The Lifesaving Nutritional Program Based on the Diet of the Island of Crete,* (New York: HarperCollins Publishers, 1975).

10. Facts from the CDC (Center for Disease Control). www.cdc.gov/nccdphp/dnpa/obesity/index.htm

11. Allport, *The Queen of Fats.*

12. A. P. David, A. J. Hulbert, and L. H. Storlien, "Dietary Fats, Membrane Phospholipids and Obesity," *The Journal of Nutrition* (1993).

13. H. O. Bang, J. Dyerberg, A. B. Nielsen, "Plasma lipid and lipoprotein pattern in Greenlandic West-coast Eskimos," *The Lancet,* no. 1 (1971).

14. William E. M. Lands, "Fish, Omega-3 And Human Health," *American Oil Chemists Society* (2005).

15. Allport, *The Queen of Fats.*

16. Allport, *The Queen of Fats.*

17. www.hsph.harvard.edu/nutritionsource/questions/omega-3/index.html

18. Allport, *The Queen of Fats.*

19. C. Gerson, B. Bishop, J. Shwed, and R. Stone, *Healing the Gerson Way: Defeating Cancer and Other Chronic Diseases* (Carmel: Totality Books, 2007).

20. Simopoulos, *The Omega Diet*
21. www.nutritiondata.com
22. Allport, *The Queen of Fats.*

CHAPTER 17
1. Flora Van Orden, *Conversations with Dr. Flora,* 2005, http://TheRawDiet.com.

SELECTED BIBLIOGRAPHY

Albi, Johnna, and Catherine Walthers. *Greens Glorious Greens!* New York: St. Martin's Press, 1996.

Appleton, Nancy. *Rethinking Pasteur's Germ Theory.* Berkeley, CA: North Atlantic, 2002.

Baker, Elizabeth. *Unbelievably Easy Sprouting!* Poulsbo, WA: privately printed, 2000.

Baroody, Theodore A., Jr. *Alkalize or Die.* Portland, OR: Eclectic, 1991.

Brown, Ellen, J. D. Hodgson, and Richard T. Hansen. *The Key to Ultimate Health.* 2nd ed. Fullerton, CA: Advanced Health Research, 2000.

Campbell, T. Colin. *The China Study.* Dallas: BenBella, 2004.

Cooper, Kenneth H. *Advanced Nutritional Therapies.* Nashville: Thomas Nelson, 1996.

Cutrell, Doug, and Ann Wigmore. *Living Foods Manual.* San Fidel, NM: privately printed.

Feldt, Linda Diane. *Spinach and Beyond.* Ann Arbor, MI: Moon Field, 2003.

Fouts, Roger. *Next of Kin.* New York: HarperCollins, 2003.

Fuhrman, Joel. *Eat to Live: The Revolutionary Formula for Fast and Sustained Weight Loss.* New York: Little Brown, 2003.

Gebhardt, Susan E., and Robin G. Thomas. *Nutritive Value of Foods.* Rev. ed. Washington, DC: U.S. Government Printing Office, 2002.

Goodall, Jane. *The Chimpanzees of Gombe.* Cambridge, MA: Belknap, 1986.

———. *Reason for Hope.* New York: Warner, 1999.

———. *Through a Window.* Boston: Houghton Mifflin, 1990.

Harris, Ben Charles. *Eat the Weeds.* Norwalk, CT: Keats, 1973.

Jensen, Bernard. *Come Alive!* Escondido, CA: Bernard Jensen, 1997.

———. *Tissue Cleansing through Bowel Management.* Escondido, CA: Bernard Jensen, 1981.

Kliment, Felicia Drury. *The Acid Alkaline Balance Diet.* New York: Contemporary, 2002.

Krishnamurti, Jiddu. *Think on These Things.* New York: Harper and Row, 1964.

Ladygina-Kohts, N. N. *Infant Chimpanzee and Human Child.* New York: Oxford University Press, 2002.

Ley, Beth M. *Flax! Fabulous Flax!* Hanover, MN: BL, 2003.

Mindell, Earl. *Food as Medicine.* New York: Simon and Schuster, 1994.

Peterson, Lee Allen. *Edible Wild Plants.* New York: Houghton Mifflin, 1977.

Price, Weston A. *Nutrition and Physical Degeneration.* 6th ed. Lemon Grove, CA: Price-Pottenger Nutrition Foundation, 2003.

Ragnar, Peter. *How Long Do You Choose to Live?* Asheville, NC: Roaring Lion, 2001.

Ross, Julia. *The Diet Cure.* New York: Penguin, 1999.

Ruimerman, Ronald. *Modeling and Remodeling in Bone Tissue.* Eindhoven, Netherlands: Eindhoven University Press, 2005.

Seibold, Ronald L. *Cereal Grass.* Lawrence, KS: Pines International, 2003.

Shahani, Khem. *Cultivate Health from Within.* Ridgefield, CT: Vital Health, 2005.

Stanway, Andrew. *The High-Fiber Diet Book.* New York: Exeter, 1976.

Tompkins, Peter, and Christopher Bird. *The Secret Life of Plants.* New York: Harper and Row, 1989.

———. *Secrets of the Soil.* Anchorage: Earthpulse, 2002.

Tooshi, Alan M. *Dr. Tooshi's High Fiber Diet.* Lincoln, NE: iUniverse.com, 2001.

Van Orden, Flora. *Conversations with Dr. Flora.* http://TheRawDiet.com, 2005.

Wigmore, Ann. *Overcoming AIDS.* New York: Copen, 1987.

———. *Rebuild Your Health.* San Fidel, NM: Ann Wigmore Foundation, 1991.

———. *You Are the Light of the World.* San Fidel, NM: Ann Wigmore Foundation, 1990.

Wigmore, Ann, and G. H. Earp-Thomas. *Organic Soil.* Boston: Rising Sun, 1978.

Wigmore, Ann, and Lee Pattinson. *The Blending Book.* New York: Avery, 1997.

Winick, Myron. *The Fiber Prescription.* New York: Ballantine, 1992.

Young, Robert O., and Shelly Redford. *The pH Miracle.* New York: Warner, 2002.

INDEX

Index

Index

Jensen, Bernard, 49, 57, 81
Joy for Life retreat, 129, 133
juicing, 16, 51–52

kale, 21, 28, 55, 93, 121, 124
   amino acid content in, 42, 43
   Green Delicious Smoothie, 187
   nutritional content of, 35, 36
   Nutritiously Bitter Smoothie, 187
   Sergei's Favorite Smoothie, 186
   Two-Layer Pudding, 190
   used in green smoothies, 177, 180,
     182, 186, 191
kidneys, 119, 120, 122, 140
Kiwi Enjoyment Smoothie, 181
Komaki, Hisatoki, 84
Korolkov, P. A., 84
kumquats, Spinach Kumquat Paradise
   Pudding, 190–191

lambsquarters, 36, 42, 43, 94
   Raw Family Wild Banango, 178
   Weeds for Kids Smoothie, 180–181
Lands, William E. M., 101
lemon, 178, 182–183, 184–185, 189, 191
   Orion's Lemon Jalapeño Smoothie, 186
lentils, 107
lethargy, 117, 128
lettuce, cos or romaine. See romaine or cos
   lettuce
lettuce, green leaf. See green leaf lettuce
lettuce, red leaf. See red leaf lettuce
lime, 176, 177, 181, 184, 185, 186–187, 190
lipoprotein (LDL), 78
Litman, Burton, 102
litmus paper, 79–80
liver cleansing, 87, 86
liver spots, 140
living foods, 114
Living Light Culinary Institute, 130
low stomach acidity, 65–66
   See also stomach acid

mallow (Malva), 177
mangoes, 55, 176, 178, 180

Mango-Parsley Pudding, 191
   Weeds for Kids Smoothie, 180–181
marathon runner, 136–137
Mediterranean Green Smoothie, 184
menstruation, 87, 117
Merry Grasshopper Smoothie, 178
metabolism, 97, 101–102
microorganisms in soil, 81–83, 88, 92
minerals, 36, 62, 82
mint, 188, 191
Minti-Dandelion Smoothie, 177
Minty Thrill Smoothie, 182
moles, 23
mood swings, 121
Mosséri, Albert, 52
mustard greens, Mustard-Cilantro Soup,
   184–185

nails, condition of, 23, 25, 72, 119, 127
National Nutritional Database, 37
neurotransmitters, 45
Nigerians and fatty acids, 102–103
nighttime eating, 18, 24
nutritional content of greens, 27–32
   lack of research/data regarding, 35, 42
   and protein, 41–47
nutritional research, 4–5
Nutritiously Bitter Smoothie, 187
nuts, 16, 104, 110–111

oats, 107
obesity, 99, 100–101, 129–130
   See also weight gain; weight loss
observation as key to learning, 1–5
"Ode to Green Smoothie," 25–26
oils, 16, 99, 101, 103–104, 105
olive oil, 105
omega-3 fatty acids, 54, 97–111
   conversion into DHA or EPA, 102
   flexibility of, 98
   greens found in, 102–103
   human deficiency in, 100
   and omega-6s, food charts of ratios
     between, 105–109
   rapid rancidity of, 103

Victoria Boutenko is an author, teacher, inventor, researcher, art-
ist, and mother of three. In 1994, when the Boutenko family, also
known as the Raw Family, became seriously ill, she sought out alternative health paths and discovered the raw food lifestyle, which enabled the family to achieve vibrant health.

Now Boutenko travels all over the world sharing her inspiring
story and teaching classes on the raw-food diet. Using the latest
scientific research, she explains the numerous benefits of choosing
a diet of raw rather than cooked foods and the importance of consuming large amounts of leafy greens. Boutenko's most recent and
powerful contribution to our understanding of dietary needs is her
research on the nutritional value of greens and her development of
green smoothies, which have revolutionized the way people access
health, no matter what their diet or lifestyle.